In Clinical P

For further volumes:
http://www.springer.com/series/13483

Jo Howard • Paul Telfer

Sickle Cell Disease in Clinical Practice

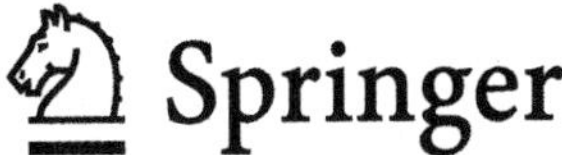

Jo Howard
Department of Haematology
Guy's and St Thomas' Hospital
London
UK

Paul Telfer
Department of Haematology
Royal London Hospital
London
UK

ISSN 2199-6652 ISSN 2199-6660 (electronic)
ISBN 978-1-4471-2472-6 ISBN 978-1-4471-2473-3 (eBook)
DOI 10.1007/978-1-4471-2473-3
Springer London Heidelberg New York Dordrecht

Library of Congress Control Number: 2014956017

Printed on acid-free paper

Springer is part of Springer Science+Business Media (www.springer.com)

Foreword

Sickle cell disease (SCD) is now one of the most common genetic condition seen in the UK with numbers increasing on an annual basis. In the 1970s, patients were limited almost entirely to London and other large cities, but now there is a reasonable expectation that patients will present with sickle cell crisis and complications in acute hospitals or general practice anywhere in the UK. SCD is an issue also for clinicians practising in almost any specialty, as it is not only a multi-organ condition which may affect the brain, kidneys, eyes or lungs, but in addition, it can complicate the presentation of other acute or chronic medical conditions. All doctors and nurses should therefore have a working knowledge of the common complications of SCD and how to treat them.

This book, written by two haematologists with large sickle practices and extensive experience of looking after patients with SCD, aims to provide this information in a well-structured and easy to read format. It deals with the acute and chronic complications of SCD and also provides guidance on providing outpatient care and on provision of care in special circumstances such as pregnancy and peri-operative management. It will be useful for haematologists, acute physicians and general practitioners who may look after these patients on a regular basis. It will also be an excellent resource for specialists who may only occasionally see patients with SCD but need to find out more about the disease in relation to their own specialties.

Dame Sally Davies
Chief Medical Officer for England
Formerly Director General for
Research and Development
National Health Service, UK

Professor of Haemoglobinopathies
Imperial College London, UK

Preface

Sickle-cell disease (SCD) is now a common condition in the UK and other European countries. This is a consequence of the recent influx of immigrants from parts of the world where the sickle-cell gene has persisted at high frequency, particularly Sub-Saharan Africa. In England the birth rate for SCD is about 1 in 2,000 new births, which is the highest rate for any inherited condition. Overall, there are about 15,000 patients living with SCD in England, and their health care needs are increasing year by year. The number of acute hospital admissions and planned episodes of care are 50 % higher than a decade ago.

SCD is a challenging condition to manage, requiring a combination of clinical expertise and experience as well as sensitivity to social and cultural context. There are acute and long-term complications which are unique to SCD and affect nearly every system of the body. Psychological co-morbidities compound the physical disorder and contribute to a reduced quality of life and probably also to reduced life expectancy. While recognising the severity of the problems, it is encouraging to note that there have been significant recent advances in understanding its pathophysiology, and several well-conducted randomized controlled trials have provided an evidence base for treatment.

Health care resources for SCD in the UK are acknowledged to be inadequate, and health care professionals, particularly those working in lower-prevalence areas, often lack the required clinical experience.

Our aim in writing this book is to promote higher-quality care. It is written from a UK perspective based on our experience in managing very large pediatric and adult specialized centres in London and witnessing our patients growing up and growing older. We hope it will also be a useful reference for those working in other countries in the developed and developing world. Our intended target audience includes medical students, general physicians, general practitioners, hematologists, pediatricians, nurse specialists and commissioners.

We have organized the text into sections covering problems as they arise in clinical practice, and have attempted to cover essential background information including up-to-date research and useful points to guide management. We have tried to deal with pediatric and adult issues in the same section wherever possible, reflecting our belief that SCD should be managed as a lifelong condition with variations in its manifestations at stages of life but reflecting the same underlying pathophysiology. In addition, we have generally not separated the sections according to genotype as the majority of complications are seen in all genotypes, albeit in differing frequencies.

We hope that this book will be a useful resource for students and heatlh care workers, and will help to promote a better understanding of SCD.

London, UK

Jo Howard
Paul Telfer

Bibliography

Modell B, Darlison M. Global epidemiology of hemoglobin disorders and derived service indicators. Bull World Health Organ. 2008;86(6):480–7.

National Hemoglobinopathy Registry. www.nhr.nhs.uk.

NCEPOD. 'A Sickle Crisis.' A report of the National Confidential Enquiry into Patient Outcome and Death 2008. http://www.ncepod.org.uk.2008sc.htm.

NHS Screening Programmes Sickle Cell and Thalassemia. Data Report 2012/3. Trends and performance analysis. www.sct.screening.nhs.uk.

Overview Report – SC&T 2010/11 Peer Review Programme. www.wmqrs.nhs.uk/reviewprogrammes/view/sickle-cell-and-thalassaemia-children. 1/9/2011.

Overview Report – 2012/13 Adults with Hemoglobin Disorders reviews. www.wmqrs.nhs.uk/reviewprogrammes/view/adults-with-hemoglobin-disorders. 4/9/2013.

Sickle cell disease in childhood. Standards and guidelines for clinical care. 2nd ed. 2010. www.sct.screening.nhs.uk.

Standards for the Clinical Care of Adults with Sickle Cell Disease in the UK. Sickle Cell Society 2008. www.sicklecellsociety.

Acknowledgements

We would like to thank the following for their helpful suggestions on improving the manuscript. Any inconsistencies or errors which remain are the fault of the authors. Thank you to Marcus Bankes, Satyajit Bhattacharya, Shohreh Beski, Cormac Breen, Frank Chinegwundoh, Yvonne Daniel, Josu De La Fuente, Jane Evanson, Graham Foster, Simon Gibbs, Nicholas Hart, Carolyn Hemsley, Banu Kaya, Rachel Kesse-Adu, Fenella Kirkham, Sebastian Lucas, Fred Piel, Esther Posner, Mira Razzak, Ashwin Reddy, Alison Thomas. We would also like to thank our families for their support: Thank you to Matthew, Jack, Adam, Chris and Pauline, Danae, Harry, Alex, John, Anne, Trevor.

Contents

Part I
General Principles of Pathophysiology, Diagnosis and Management

Chapter 1
Overview of Sickle Cell Disease

Introduction

In this section, we describe the structure and function of the haemoglobin molecule, red blood cells and blood vessels. This is not a comprehensive account, but will help in understanding the principles as they relate to sickle cell disease.

Basic Physiology

Hemoglobin

The hemoglobin molecule is composed of four subunits each of which contains a protein chain (globin), which encloses a flat ring-like molecular structure (the heme prosthetic group) where oxygen is bound. Hemoglobin has been refined through evolution and is the central player in a system of molecules, biochemical reactions and biological compartments whose integrity is essential for gas exchange. The process involves uptake of oxygen in the alveolar beds of the lungs, where concentration (measured as partial pressure) is high, and release in the tissues, where concentration is low. Simultaneously, carbon dioxide is taken up in the tissues and released in the lungs.

J. Howard, P. Telfer, *Sickle Cell Disease in Clinical Practice*, In Clinical Practice, DOI 10.1007/978-1-4471-2473-3_1,

When oxygen binds to a heme subunit, there is change in the shape of the hemoglobin molecule, due to interactions with amino acids in the adjacent globin chain. This facilitates binding at the other heme subunits within the tetramer and promotes oxygen carriage. These interactions are affected by amino acid substitutions in the globin chain.

Hemoglobin is compartmentalized within the red blood cell and if released into the circulation as free hemoglobin is not able to participate in effective gas exchange. Free hemoglobin may cause circulatory and renal toxicity, through binding and inactivating nitric oxide, a small molecule which has an important role in controlling blood flow (principally through its effects on the vessel wall).

This compartmentalization of hemoglobin within the red cell also enables it to play a major role in carbon dioxide transport, through buffering hydrogen ions produced from the conversion of carbon dioxide and water to bicarbonate and hydrogen ions.

2,3-biphosphoglycerate (2,3-BPG) is an important by-product of the breakdown of glucose (glycolysis) within the red blood cell and interacts with hemoglobin to facilitate oxygen delivery by shifting the oxygen dissociation curve to the right. When oxygen concentration in the tissues is low, and metabolism of glucose are predominantly anaerobic rather than aerobic, excess lactic acid is produced, and this results in increased intra-erythrocytic 2,3 DPG.

Hemoglobin is synthesized in red cell precursors (erythroblasts) during their differentiation within the bone marrow, and continues to be synthesized in the cytoplasm of the youngest population of circulating red cells, the reticulocytes. Mature red cells lack the enzymes and organelles required for its continued synthesis.

Iron destined for heme synthesis is transported to the erythron in its oxidized (ferric, Fe^{3+}) state bound to plasma transferrin (Tf). Erythroblasts express plentiful transferrin receptors on their surface, and these can bind the iron-Tf complex, leading to internalization by endocytosis. Intracellular mobilization of iron occurs through a pathway consisting of acidification of the interior of the endosome, release and reduction of iron to its ferrous (Fe^{2+}) state, and transportation of Fe^{2+} across the endosomal membrane into the cytoplasm and subsequently into the mitochondrion via the transport protein mitoferrin. Within the mitochondrion, Fe^{2+} iron is finally incorporated into heme as the last step of heme biosynthesis, in a reaction catalysed by the enzyme ferrochelatase. Heme is then transported back into the cytoplasm for incorporation into hemoglobin.

Molecular Genetics

The beta globin cluster on Chromosome 11 consists of an array of genes encoding the beta–like globins. The alpha globin gene cluster is physically separated on chromosome 16. It differs in its genetic organization, but is regulated in concert with the beta globin cluster to ensure co-ordinated expression of the correct genes. Sequential expression of alpha-like and beta-like genes at different stages of development ensures that specific hemoglobin is produced according to the needs of the developing embryo, fetus or infant. Fetal hemoglobin is the predominant hemoglobin from about 12 weeks of gestation up until birth. It consists of two alpha and two gamma globin chains (HbF, $\alpha_2\gamma_2$) and has enhanced oxygen affinity compared to adult hemoglobin (HbA, $\alpha_2\beta_2$). This ensures that oxygen is transported efficiently across the placental membrane from HbA containing maternal red cells into HbF containing fetal red cells.

The control of expression of the globin gene clusters during development has been the subject of sustained genetic research over the past four decades. The incentive has been partly because globin gene expression is seen as a paradigm for the understanding of gene expression. Also, research has informed therapeutic approaches to managing hemoglobin disorders through gene therapy or reactivation of developmental globin gene expression in order to circumvent the genetic changes affecting adult hemoglobin (HbA).

The Sickle Mutation

The mutation is a C to A substitution at codon 6 of the beta globin gene, which results in a substitution of the neutral amino acid valine for glutamic acid. The sickle hemoglobin molecule is designated HbS ($\alpha_2\beta^s_2$).

The Sickling Process

In the deoxygenated state, HbS molecules form a polymeric structure where individual molecules stack up into fibres, and then aggregate into a rope-like structure of inter-twined fibre-pairs. When hemoglobin becomes oxygenated, the array denatures. The structure is formed though non-covalent interactions between adjacent hemoglobin molecules. This is made possible through exposure of binding sites during the process of oxygenation and deoxygenation of HbS. Molecules are stabilized in this polymeric structure because of a new interaction between the substituted β6 valine and a neutral pocket on adjacent hemoglobin molecules. The normal glutamic acid residue at position 6 of beta globin cannot participate in this interaction because of its shape and charge (Fig. 1.1).

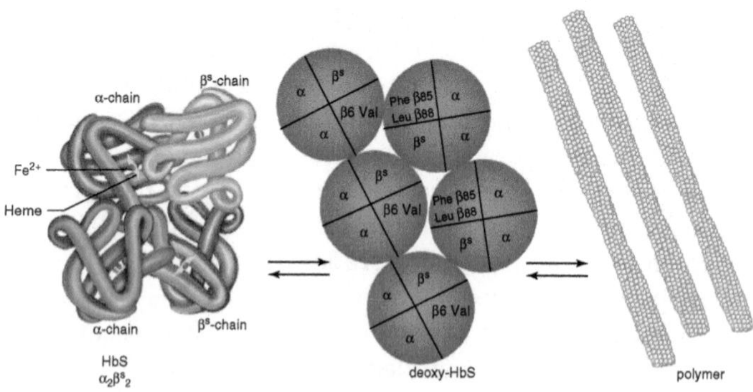

FIGURE 1.1 The sickling process. The hemoglobin molecule, comprising four globin chains each with a heme group, is shown on the *left*. The sickle mutation results in a valine substitution at position 6 of the beta globin chain. This is able to form a new interaction with amino acids at positions 85 and 88 of adjacent beta globin chains when hemoglobin is in the deoxygenated state. Multiplication of these interactions leads to propagation of sickle hemoglobin polymers

The time lag from deoxygenation of hemoglobin to polymer formation enables the red cell to traverse the capillary bed and return to the lungs for uptake of oxygen, whereupon the polymer can deaggregate. This sickling/desickling cycle is repeated with each circulation of the red cell. If retarded, extensive polymerization of hemoglobin can occur before returning to the alveolar beds, resulting in red cell damage. The potential for a damaging positive feedback of more obstruction leading to more sickling can easily be appreciated.

Several factors influence the speed of polymer formation:

1. *Intracellular hemoglobin concentration.* Higher mean corpuscular hemoglobin concentration (MCHC) facilitates sickling. Lower MCHC (e.g. with co-inheritance of alpha thalassemia, or concomitant iron deficiency) retards sickling.
2. *Presence of other intracellular hemoglobins.* Some hemoglobins (e.g. HbA, HbF) inhibit sickling, and some hemoglobin variants (HbC, HbD^{Punjab}, HbO^{Arab}) are permissive. These interactions explain why carriers of sickle cell (HbAS) and double heterozygotes with hereditary persistence of fetal hemoglobin (HbS/HPFH) are protected against sickling, while some double heterozygotes (e.g. HbSC, $HbSD^{Punjab}$, $HbSO^{Arab}$) have a clinically significant sickle condition.
3. *Intracellular pH and temperature.* Low pH and a raised temperature increase sickling in vitro, and may also play a role in clinical situations. These may be part of the explanation for onset of acute crisis associated with fever and conditions of acidosis.

Consequences of Sickling

Erythrocytic Damage

Intracellular sickling of hemoglobin can damage the red cell through several inter-related mechanisms, all leading to reduced red cell survival (hemolysis)

1. *Damage to the membrane and cytoskeleton.* Red cells are adapted to squeeze through narrow diameter blood vessels

(the narrowest capillary vessels are about one third of the red cell diameter). This is made possible by the elasticity of the protein matrix arranged underneath the cell membrane (the cytoskeleton). Extensive polymer formation and repetitive cycles of sickling and de-sickling eventually result in irreversible damage to the membrane and cytoskeleton, giving rise to irreversibly sickled cells (ISC's). An increase in circulating ISC count is associated with enhanced hemolysis but not with frequency of vaso-occlusive crises.

2. *Changes in the red cell membrane.* Damage to the cell membrane and cytoskeleton also results in the expression of adhesive cell surface molecules, and increased exposure of negatively charged phospholipid on the red cell surface, leading to enhanced adherence to the vascular endothelium.
3. *Red cell dehydration.* Erythrocytes containing sickle hemoglobin, particularly reticulocytes and ISC's, can become dehydrated, with an increase in mean intra-corpuscular hemoglobin concentration (MCHC). This is independent of the state of hydration of the body as a whole. Sickling of hemoglobin enhances loss of water and electrolytes and potentiates influx of calcium across the cell membrane. The Gardos channel, an important governor of ion and water exchange, is activated by increased intracellular calcium and mediates loss of potassium ions and water. It is known to be activated in SCD erythrocytes, and has been seen as a possible therapeutic target.
4. *Impaired anti-oxidant mechanisms.* Maintenance of hemoglobin in its reduced state, and protection of the erythrocyte against the toxic effects of denatured hemoglobin and unbound heme requires an intact system of intracellular anti-oxidant pathways, and these are also impaired in SCD erythrocytes.

Vaso-Occlusion (Fig. 1.2)

Experimental systems have been developed to visualize the process of vaso-occlusion, making use of transgenic mice

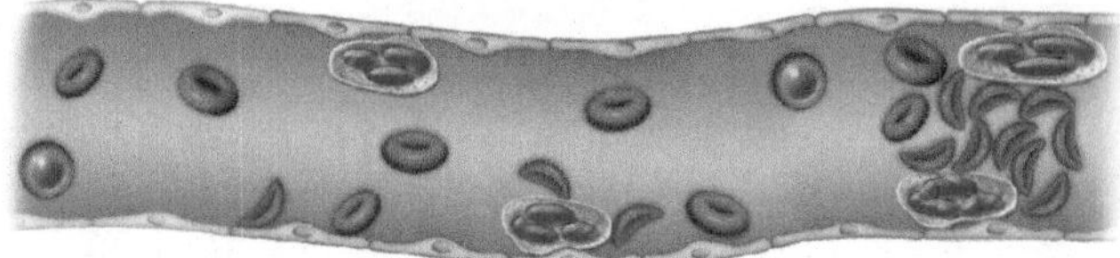

FIGURE 1.2 Blood cell and endothelial interactions leading to vaso-occlusion

expressing exclusively human sickle hemoglobin. Vaso-occlusion can be induced by the inflammatory process which occurs when a viewing chamber is inserted surgically to observe the microvascular flow in these animals. This is greatly accentuated by injecting inflammatory cytokines such as tumour necrosis factor (TNF). These activate a whole cascade of effectors (leucocytes, endothelium, platelets, coagulation factors) implicated in the process of vaso-occlusion. An important early event is adhesion of HbS-containing erythrocytes to the vessel wall, either directly to the endothelium, or indirectly, through binding to adherent, activated neutrophils. This results in a log-jam of erythrocytes which occlude flow, leading to ischemia, infarction, and subsequent reperfusion injury (Figs. 1.2 and 1.3). Characterization of ligands and receptors involved in these adhesive interactions and the events involved in cellular activation are leading to development of anti-sickling drugs which attenuate the clinical effects of vaso-occlusion.

Nitric Oxide Depletion

Nitric oxide (NO) is a small molecule which has an important function in controlling local blood flow. It is produced in the

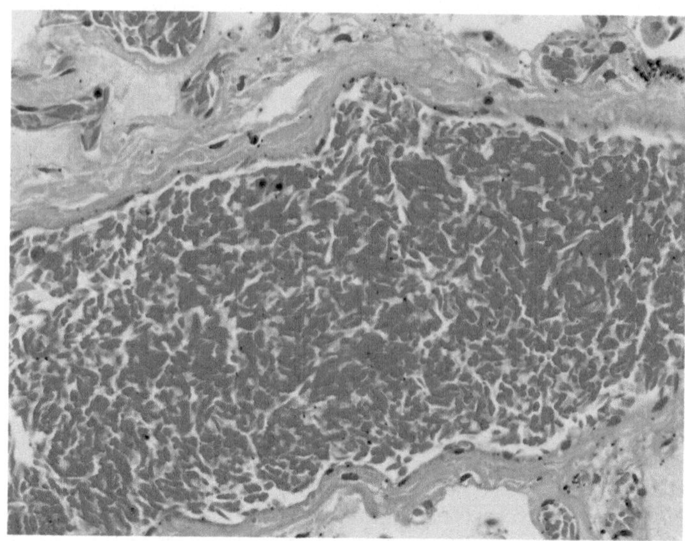

FIGURE 1.3 Histological specimen of the lung from a fatal case of acute chest syndrome showing occlusion of a medium sized pulmonary vessel with sickled erythrocytes

endothelium from the amino acid L-arginine in a reaction catalysed by nitric oxide synthase (NOS). One form of this enzyme catalyses a constant background production, whilst a further inducible form catalyses a higher rate of production in response to endothelial activation. NO diffuses from the endothelium into underlying smooth muscle cells and causes relaxation of smooth muscle, vasodilatation and increased blood flow.

Depletion of NO is an important cause of circulatory disturbance and vascular damage in SCD. Proposed mechanisms for this include breakdown of sickled erythrocytes within the vessel lumen (intravascular hemolysis). This releases free hemoglobin to scavenge NO and also causes diversion of NO to detoxify antioxidants produced from degraded hemoglobin.

Inflammation and Tissue Damage

The pathway to tissue damage in SCD is likely to involve endothelial activation, adhesion and activation of leukocytes, together with free-radical generation from interaction of NO with free plasma hemoglobin, release of heme from degraded intravascular hemoglobin, and hypoxia-reperfusion injury. Figure 1.4 illustrates how these mechanisms can interact and form a positive feedback loop, leading to more vaso-occlusion and more tissue damage.

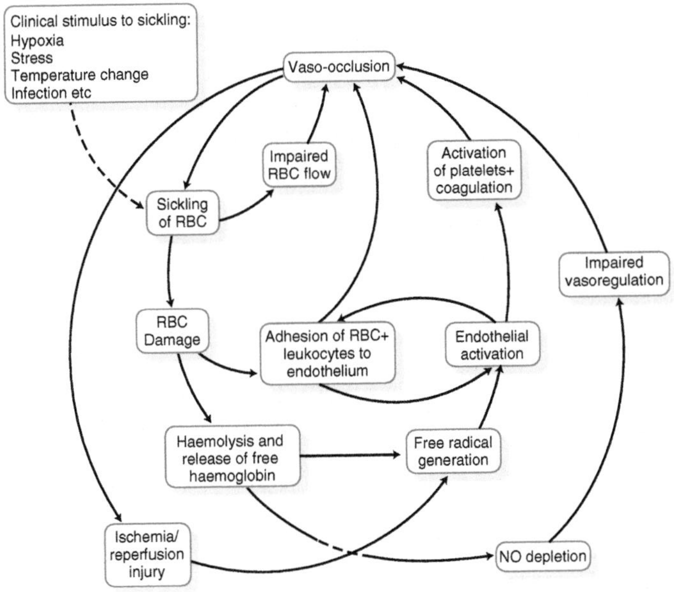

FIGURE 1.4 Pathophysiological processes involved in vaso-occlusion

New Treatments

There is a profusion of new drugs in development for the treatment of SCD which exploit the mechanisms outlined above. Some of these are listed in Table 1.1. It is unlikely that one drug will be effective in controlling the entire process, and future trials will probably exploit combinations of drugs acting synergistically at different stages of the process of vaso-occlusion.

TABLE 1.1 Potential drugs for treatment of SCD and their mechanism of action

Mechanism	Drug
HbF induction	Hydroxyurea
	Pomalidomide
	Butyrate analogues
Gardos channel inhibition	Senicapoc
Nitric oxide replenishment	Inhaled nitric oxide
	L-Arginine
Hemoxygenase induction	MP4CO
Intravascular hemolysis	Haptoglobin
Inhibition of endothelial adhesion	GMI 1070
	Intravenous immunoglobulins
	Heparin
Inhibition of red cell adhesion	Propranolol
Inhibition of platelet adhesion	Prasugrel

Pathological Effects of Sickling

These cellular and local circulatory disturbances can provoke a variety of pathological processes as described below. How these affect the different organs and systems will be described in subsequent sections.

Although SCD is highly variable in severity it can be helpful to envisage a spectrum of clinical phenotypes ranging from hemolytic at one end (characterized by severe anemia, high cardiac output, pulmonary hypertension and ankle ulceration) to vaso-occlusive (higher steady state hemoglobin, frequent acute pain crises and acute chest syndrome) at the other end of the spectrum.

Sequestration

Sequestration refers to the trapping of a large mass of erythrocytes, resulting in worsening of anemia and, if severe, circulatory collapse. This occurs in highly vascular organs which have a capacity to expand. The spleen is particularly susceptible because its circulation involves passage of red cells through endothelial fenestrations (small gaps) into splenic sinusoids, where redundant red cell membrane and cellular inclusions are removed by sinus macrophages (Fig. 1.5). For HbS-containing red cells, reduced flexibility impairs passage through the fenestrations. This is followed by impaired flow through the sinusoids. The result is an increase in intracellular sickling, erythrocytic damage and vascular obstruction. It is not surprising that the spleen is the first organ to become dysfunctional. Sequestered cells are not necessarily permanently damaged, and clinical experience suggests that they

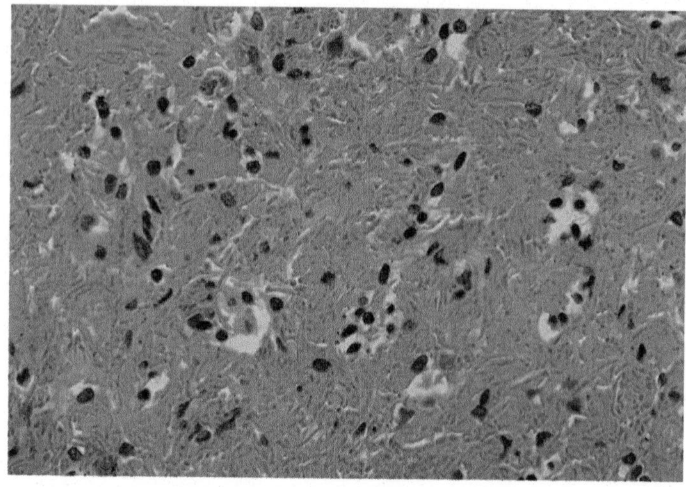

FIGURE 1.5 Acute splenic sequestration. Histological section of postmortem spleen from a patient with HbSS showing intense sinusoidal congestion with sickled *red* cells

can re-enter the circulation (auto-transfusion). Sequestration also contributes to acute liver damage (acute hepatic sequestration), acute chest syndrome and priapism.

Hemolytic Anemia

Hemolysis is the term used to describe shortened red cell survival. When hemolysis results in reduced hemoglobin concentration, with inadequate bone marrow capacity to keep pace with red cell loss, this is referred to as hemolytic anemia. The normal mean survival of a red cell is 120 days, and this is reduced to 10 days or less in HbSS. Damaged and effete red cells are normally removed from the circulation by reticulo-endothelial macrophages in the spleen, liver and bone marrow. This is also the predominant mechanism for red cell removal in SCD (extravascular hemolysis), however, about one third of hemolysis in SCD is due to lysis of red cells within the circulation as a consequence of rupture of red blood cell membrane (intravascular hemolysis). This results in release of free hemoglobin into the circulation, which is toxic. Free hemoglobin can be scavenged and transported to reticulo-endothelial macrophages in a non-toxic form bound to the plasma protein haptoglobin. Free heme is similarly transported bound to hemopexin. Plasma levels of haptoglobin and hemopexin are reduced and can be overwhelmed in steady state and during acute crisis of SCD. Other abnormalities associated with hemolysis include an increase in serum bilirubin (from breakdown of heme) and elevated serum levels of the enzyme lactate dehydrogenase (LDH) which is released from damaged RBC's. The bone marrow responds to increased red cell breakdown by accelerating red cell production, with a consequent increased release of young red cells (reticulocytes) into the circulation.

The rate of hemolysis is typically higher in HbSS than in other genotypes but there is variability from one individual to another, partly explained by known genetic modifiers such as hereditary persistence of fetal hemoglobin, and co-inheritance of alpha thalassemia. Hemolysis is accelerated during acute vaso-occlusive crises, infections and episodes of sequestration. In Africa, children with SCD infected with malaria may hemolyse at an increased rate and develop profound anemia.

Microvascular Occlusion

The pathophysiology of vaso-occlusion in the microcirculation (arteriole, capillary and post-capillary venule) has already been described. The consequences include ischemia, infarction, reperfusion injury, inflammation and tissue damage. Microvascular occlusion is thought to be an important mechanism underlying the development of acute painful crisis and acute chest syndrome.

Large Vessel Lesions

A variety of vascular lesions affect the arterial side of the circulation. These probably result from long-term endothelial damage brought about by adherent RBC's and shearing of sickled RBC's at high flow rate. The characteristic sites are points of turbulence (e.g. arterial bifurcations). Chronic endothelial injury results in changes to the underlying vessel wall, loss of elastic lamina, fibrosis and smooth muscle proliferation. The characteristic lesions seen in the large cerebral arteries (vascular stenoses, and aneurysm formation) are probably the end-results of this process. Stenotic lesions have also been reported in pulmonary and splenic arteries.

Neovascularization is another process seen in SCD, associated with chronic ischemia and arterial occlusion or stenosis. The two most familiar examples of this are sea fan neovascularization of the retina, and moyamoya formation associated with occlusion or stenosis of the terminal internal carotid artery (tICA) and proximal middle cerebral artery (MCA) and/or anterior cerebral artery (ACA).

Sickle Genotypes

Homozygous sickle cell disease (*HbSS*). This is the commonest genotype and the main focus of this book.

Hemoglobin SC disease (*HbSC*). Haemoglobin C is a haemoglobin variant in which lysine substitutes for glutamic acid at position 6 of the beta globin chain. HbC does not sickle, but is permissive to sickling of HbS. It is a common variant in West Africans (e.g. Nigerians and Ghanaians). The compound heterozygote condition HbSC is encountered frequently in these populations and is a clinically significant condition. Compared to HbSS, steady state hemoglobin levels are generally higher, acute crises are less frequent and severe, and predicted life expectancy is improved. The most common chronic complications are avascular necrosis of the hips, proliferative retinopathy, and renal tubular concentrating deficits. As with HbSS, children with HbSC are identified at birth with neonatal screening in the UK and should be entered into long-term comprehensive care programmes.

Sickle thalassemia. Beta thalassemia is characterized by decreased (β^+ thalassemia) or absent (β^0 thalassemia) production of beta globin chains. Beta thalassemia and other thalassemic alleles (e.g. Lepore, delta beta, HbE), when co-inherited with the sickle gene, result in a sickling condition of variable severity. Individuals with HbS β^+ thalassemia produce small amounts of HbA which inhibit HbS polymerization and this results in a milder clinical phenotype. Individuals with HbS β^0 thalassemia produce HbS and no HbA and have a clinical phenotype similar to HbSS.

Other sickle genotypes. Hemoglobin SD^{Punjab} and Hemoglobin SO^{Arab} are less common compound heterozygote conditions which are similar in severity to HbSS.

Clinically insignificant sickle genotypes. A large number of globin variants identified incidentally on hemoglobinopathy screening do not interact with HbS to produce clinically significant conditions. These include HbD^{Iran}, HbD^{Philadelphia}, HbJ, HbK Woolwich. Information about unusual variants can be found in larger textbooks covering disorders of hemoglobin or from the website: sct.screening.nhs.uk

General Aspects of Management of Milder Sickle Genotypes

The evidence for benefits of specific interventions is much clearer for HbSS than for other genotypes. Patients with milder genotypes should nevertheless be enrolled in a care programme, offered pneumococcal prophylaxis at least to the age of 5 years and be seen at least annually for clinical review. The risk of childhood stroke is much less and transcranial Doppler screening is not generally recommended for children with HbSC and HbS β^+ thalassemia.

Sickle Cell Carrier (Sickle Cell Trait, HbAS)

Carriers are protected against intracellular sickling because HbA and HbS are both synthesized in the developing erythroblast and in the mature red cell there is about twice as much HbA as HbS. This predominance of HbA is sufficient to inhibit sickling in all but the most extreme intracellular conditions of acidosis, dehydration and of prolonged deoxygenation. Between 18 and 25 % of the population in Sub Saharan African countries are carriers. In England, about 6,000 carrier babies are born each year (nearly 1 % of births).

The carrier state is not generally regarded as harmful but it has been associated with adverse clinical outcomes (listed in Table 1.2) and whilst it is important that genetic and hemoglobinopathy counsellors are aware of these associations, it must be emphasized that carriers do not have a serious medical condition. Information about possible risks should be conveyed carefully to avoid unnecessary alarm.

Renal complications are mainly a consequence of damage to the mechanism for concentration of urine. Generation of a high osmotic gradient and hemoconcentration within the vessels of the renal medulla (vasa recta) produce the conditions under which red cells can sickle. This results in stasis, vascular occlusion, vascular loss and infarction of medullary tissue.

The carrier state is also a risk factor for exercise-induced collapse, rhabdomyolysis and sudden death. Although these are very rare events, they have been observed in military and sports academies, where individuals have been subjected to

TABLE 1.2 Clinical disorders described in carriers of sickle cell

Condition	Etiology	Frequency	Evidence for association
Renal			
Hyposthenuria (impaired concentration of urine)	Vaso-occlusion and vascular damage in renal medulla	Common	Strong
Renal papillary necrosis and hematuira	Papillary infarction with vaso-occlusion and vascular damage in renal medulla	Rare	Strong
Medullary carcinoma	Unknown	Rare	Strong
Spleen			
Splenic infarction/ sequestration	Stasis and occlusion in splenic vasculature	Rare	Strong
Other			
Rhabdomyolysis		Rare	Moderate
Heat stroke		Rare	Moderate
Sudden death		Rare	Moderate

intense exercise while at a suboptimal level of fitness. High altitude, dehydration and concurrent febrile illness are additional predisposing conditions.

Acute splenic sequestration has been described in extremes of high altitude and dehydration.

Epidemiology

Analysis of shared polymorphisms in the sequences surrounding the beta globin gene locus (beta globin gene haplotypes) suggests that the sickle gene has spontaneously arisen in three different African ancestral populations and additionally in India. The reason for its persistence seems to be the selective advantage conferred in regions of high transmission of falciparum malaria where carriers are estimated to have about 90 % protection against episodes of severe malaria. The carrier frequency in countries of W Africa (e.g. Nigeria and Ghana) is 20–25 %, and in central Africa (e.g. Democratic Republic of Congo) is 15–20 %. The birth prevalence of SCD in these countries is expected to be 1–2 %. Globally, the estimated annual number of births with SCD is about 230,000. SCD is also very common in Arab populations in the Middle East (e.g. Saudi Arabia) and in tribal populations in India (for Datapoint distribution and maps of the mean and uncertainty in the predicted HbS allele frequency, an excellent resource can be found at http://www.thelancet.com/journals/lancet/article/PIIS0140-6736(12)61229-X/fulltext).

Although rare in North European and American endemic populations, SCD has become a common inherited condition because of forced introduction of African populations during the slave trade, and more recent immigration of people from former colonies of Britain, France, Belgium and the Netherlands. In England, there are approximately 12,000–15,000 individuals affected by SCD and 300 new births per year. There is a very uneven geographical distribution, with 70 % of patients and births in London and very low prevalence in the South West and North East and in rural areas.

Inheritance

Homozygous SCD is an autosomal recessive condition. Offspring of two carrier individuals have a 1 in 4 chance of having an affected child. Patterns of inheritance are shown in Fig. 1.6.

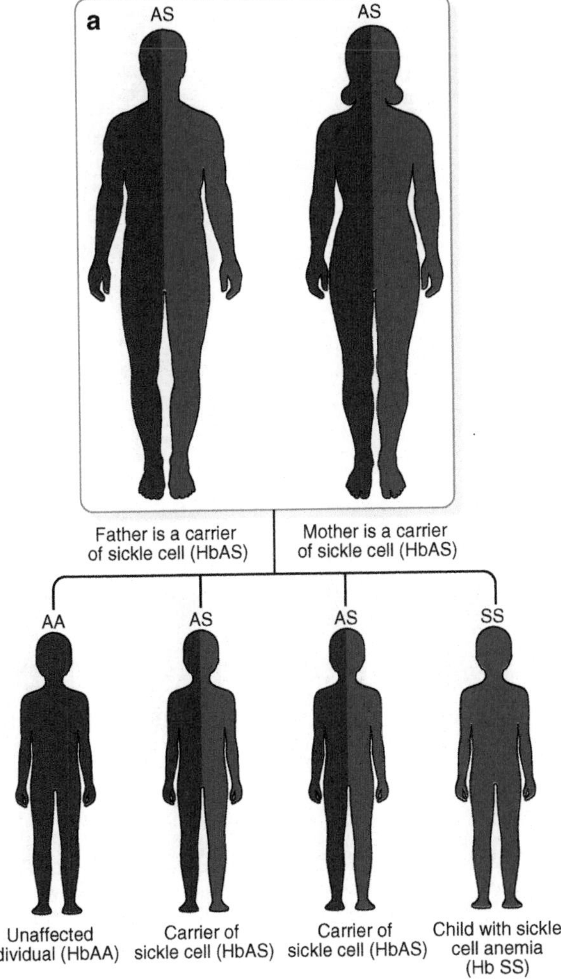

FIGURE 1.6 Inheritance diagrams (**a**) Two carrier (AS) individuals have a 1 in 4 chance of having offspring with HbSS (**b**) Two carrier individuals with different hemoglobinopathies have a 1 in 4 chance of having offspring with a compound heterozygote condition e.g. if one parent is a carrier of sickle cell and the other a carrier of beta thalassemia, there will be a 1 in 4 chance of having an affected child with HbSβ thalassemia. This will also apply to individuals who are carriers of hemoglobin C (AC), hemoglobin D-Punjab or hemoglobin E

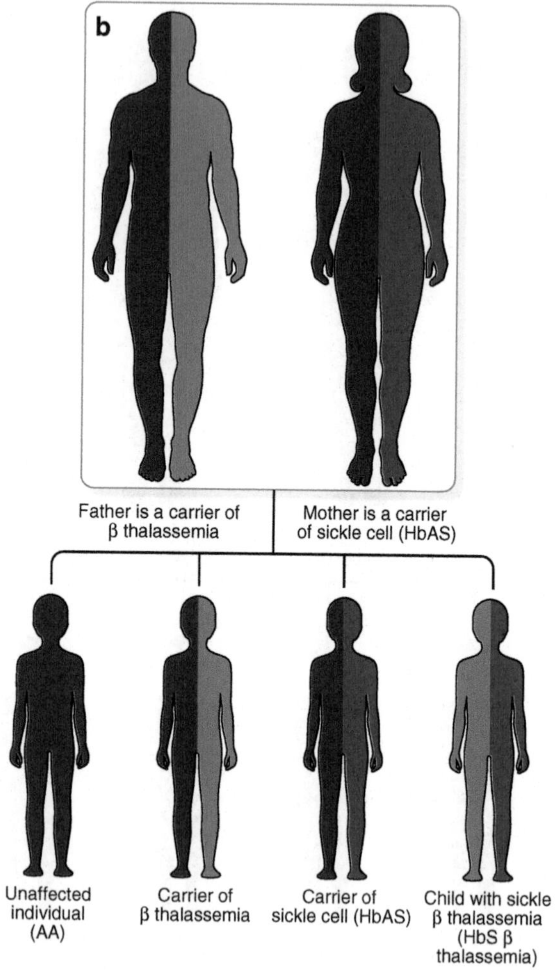

FIGURE 1.6 (continued)

Screening and Prevention of SCD

Screening is a public health activity in which individuals in a defined population are offered a test for early identification of a significant medical condition. For genetic conditions, screening programs may be may be used to identify asymptomatic carriers. Screening is justifiable if an intervention can be offered to mitigate the risk of developing the disease or the clinical consequences of the disease. Before implementation, a health economic analysis should be undertaken to demonstrate value for money. Furthermore, the ethical, sociological and cultural acceptability within the population to be screened must be carefully considered.

Targeted Versus Universal Screening

In countries where SCD is common in an ethnic minority but not in the endemic population, it may be more cost-effective to target screening, and avoid unnecessary testing of the indigenous majority population. For this to be efficient and effective, the tool(s) used to identify the at-risk minority populations must be sensitive and specific. There is further complexity because of increased population mixing between indigenous and immigrant populations. Also, information systems in the health care service may be inadequately developed to streamline the process, leading to administrative errors. The National Health Service Hemoglobinopathy Screening Programme uses a targeted approach to antenatal screening in low-prevalence areas of England.

Neonatal Screening

The aim of neonatal screening is to identify babies with SCD prior to their first clinical presentation. There is compelling evidence from programmes in Jamaica and the United States that early diagnosis can improve clinical outcomes and reduce mortality during childhood. Depending on the population, screening could be universal or targeted, but most health authorities have opted for a universal programme, partly to avoid missing an affected baby not in the at-risk population, and partly because national universal bloodspot screening programmes already exist in many developed countries (for example phenylketonuria, congenital hypothyroidism), to which SCD screening can be added relatively easily.

In the normal neonate, fetal hemoglobin predominates (usually 80–90 %) and HbA constitutes most of the remainder. In the case of a neonate with homozygous SCD, there is no HbA, and HbS is present at 10–20 % of total, a finding which is usually reported as HbF+S. It is important to note that this result is also obtained with other sickle genotypes (HbS/HPFH, HbS β^0 thalassemia, HbS $\delta\beta$ thalassemia). Knowledge of the parental carrier status is the best way of confirming the genotype, and this is one benefit of the linked antenatal and neonatal screening programme in England.

Interventions which can be offered include parental education, enrolment in a care programme, early initiation of oral penicillin, administration of pneumococcal vaccination and transcranial Doppler screening. Parental education is particularly important, and early recognition of serious crises will help to prevent infant mortality from acute complications such as invasive pneumococcal disease, acute splenic sequestration and acute chest crisis.

Screening to Identify Carriers of Sickle Cell Disease

The aims of these programmes are:

1. To make individuals aware of their carrier status
2. To enable carriers to make an informed choice about avoiding an affected birth

There is no consensus about the optimal method and timing for carrier screening. National and regional health authorities have made decisions based on a wide range of considerations including health care priorities, resources, epidemiology, customs and religious beliefs. Most would agree that it is better to screen and make people aware of their carrier status at an early stage, preferably before marriage, and certainly before becoming pregnant. There are examples of successful carrier screening programmes for school children, young adults, and prior to marriage. These are mostly in countries where the gene is common in the indigenous population. Careful consideration needs to be given to avoid stigmatization of carriers belonging either to the indigenous or to an at-risk ethnic minority population.

Antenatal Screening

Antenatal Hemoglobinopathy screening is offered to all women in England as part of routine antenatal care. Testing for sickle cell carrier status is universal in high prevalence areas (more than 1.5 babies per 10,000 births with SCD) and targeted in low prevalence areas, with risk assessed by determining the family origins of baby's mother and father using a validated questionnaire (http://sct.screening.nhs.uk/foq). Carrier mothers are counselled and the fathers invited for testing. When both parents are carriers, the pregnancy is regarded as 'at risk' (1 in 4 chance of an affected child), and prenatal diagnosis (PND) offered. The aim is to perform PND by the end of the 13th week of pregnancy, however, performance indicators for the screening programme show that at-risk pregnancies are usually identified later. This is sometimes the result of local policies for delaying antenatal booking visits until 12 weeks or to mothers reporting late with their pregnancy. The national screening programme is working with antenatal services to explore ways of ensuring earlier antenatal testing. PND is performed by DNA analysis of fetal tissue taken by chorionic villus sampling (CVS) or amniocentesis. There is a small risk of miscarriage with both procedures. Couples found to have an affected fetus require further counselling and may decide to terminate the affected pregnancy.

Pre-Conceptual Screening

Pre-conceptual screening provides couples with information about the risks of an affected birth before pregnancy and allows the couple to consider the options of pre-natal diagnosis and pre-implantation genetic diagnosis (PIGD). In PIGD, a cell is removed at the blastomere stage of embryo development (16–32 cell embryo), and the cellular DNA tested for the sickle mutation after amplification by polymerase chain reaction (PCR). Using this technique, unaffected embryos produced by In Vitro Fertilization (IVF) can be implanted. This is a complicated procedure and may involve several cycles of ovulation and IVF. Success rate (rate of live births per cycle) is approximately 30 %. PIGD is available in UK clinics approved by the Human Fertilisation and Embryo Authority (HFEA).

Life Expectancy and Causes of Death

Previously there were high rates of mortality in patients under five years of age with SCD, particularly from sepsis, and this still remains the case in much of Sub Saharan Africa. Survival rates to 18 years contemporary newborn cohort studies from the UK and the US are in the region of 95–99 %, demonstrating that SCD should no longer be considered a fatal disease during childhood in high income countries. Overall life expectancy for patients with HbSS in the US has increased from around 14 years in 1973 to about 45 years by the 1990s. Limited recent data from the US suggest that there has not been a substantial improvement in survival for adults since the late 1990s. In Jamaica, the estimated mean survival is currently in the mid 50s. There are no comparable figures from the UK at present.

Women generally live longer than men, as is the case in the general population and with many chronic conditions. There is evidence of increased of mortality rates in adolescents following transition from pediatric to adult services, and average age of death in the USA in a recent report on population death certification covering the period 1979–2005 is in the mid-30's.

Improved childhood survival is due to the combined benefits of pneumococcal prophylaxis, and comprehensive pediatric care, including awareness and early management of acute crisis in childhood (e.g. acute splenic sequestration, acute chest syndrome). The poorer results for adults in the USA may reflect the lack of universal health care provision. The situation is different in the UK which benefits from a National Health Service, where all children and adult citizens can access comprehensive care free of charge.

Recent studies of causes of death in SCD have shown increasing numbers due to cardiorespiratory and renal disease. A national study of mortality in SCD in the UK showed 46 deaths over a 2 year period. Stroke, multi-organ failure and acute chest syndrome were the major causes of death. Similar data were reported in Europe although 19 % of patients died from chronic disease complications (cirrhosis, chronic renal failure and cardiac disease).

As life expectancy continues to improve and more patients reach middle and old age, new challenges are emerging in how best to manage an aging population with increasing end organ damage and chronic health problems.

Bibliography

Gaston MH, et al. Prophylaxis with oral penicillin in children with sickle cell anemia – a randomized controlled trial. New Engl J Med. 1986;314(25):1593–9.

NCEPOD. 'A sickle crisis'. A report of the national confidential enquiry into patient outcome and death 2008. http://www.ncepod.org.uk.2008sc.htm.

Perronne V, Roberts-Harewood M, Bachir D, et al. Patterns of mortality in sickle cell disease in adults in France and England. Hematol J. 2002;3:56–60.

Quinn CT, Rogers ZR, McCavit TL, Buchanan GR. Improved survival of children and adolescents with sickle cell disease. Blood. 2010;115:3447–52.

Standards for the linked antenatal and newborn screening programme. 2nd ed. Oct 2011. www.screening.nhs.uk/sickleandthal.

Streetly A, Latinovic R, Hall K, Henthorn J. Implementation of universal newborn bloodspot screening for sickle cell disease and other clinically significant hemoglobinopathies in England: screening results for 2005–7. J Clin Pathol. 2009;62(1):26–30.

Telfer P, et al. Clinical outcomes in children with SCD living in England: a neonatal cohort in East London. Hematologica. 2007;92(7):905–12.

Zeuner D, et al. Antenatal and neonatal hemoglobinopathy screening in the UK: review and economic analysis. Health Technol Assess. 1999;3(11):i–v, 1–186.

Chapter 2
Laboratory Tests Used in Diagnosis and Monitoring

Hemoglobin

The average steady state hemoglobin (Hb) level in HbSS is about 75 g/l, but there is a wide variation, with levels ranging from 50 to 110 g/l. Lower steady state values may be seen in patients with splenomegaly, high hemolytic rate, or renal impairment. Higher levels are seen with co-inheritance of alpha thalassemia, and high fetal hemoglobin (HbF). Patients with the genotypes HbSC and HbS β^+ thalassemia are mildly anemic in steady state (Hb 90–120 g/l). There is also significant variation with age. In HbSS patients, Hb levels decrease during the first few months of life and may not reach a stable steady state until the age of 2–5 years. Thereafter, they are fairly stable during childhood up to puberty, when there is an increase, particularly in males, probably because higher testosterone levels stimulate an increase in red cell mass. There is a gradual reduction after the fourth decade, partly related to deteriorating renal function.

Steady state hemoglobin level should be measured every year. This helps in assessing the significance of a drop in hemoglobin level during an acute crisis. It also gives some indication of long-term morbidity and mortality. Higher Hb levels are associated with an increased tendency to acute painful crisis and acute chest syndrome. More severe hemolytic anemia (Hb <75 g/l) is associated with a spectrum

J. Howard, P. Telfer, *Sickle Cell Disease in Clinical Practice*, In Clinical Practice, DOI 10.1007/978-1-4471-2473-3_2,

of long-term complications related to chronic hemolysis, including stroke and pulmonary hypertension.

Red Cell Indices

Red cell indices include mean cell volume (MCV) and mean cell hemoglobin (MCH). These are usually normal in HbSS. In HbSC, MCV and MCH may be normal or decreased. Low MCV and MCH (microcytic, hypochromic indices) are characteristic of HbS β thalassemia, and HbSS with co-inherited alpha thalassemia.

Red Cell Appearances on Blood Film

The characteristic features in HbSS, HbSC and HbS β^{o} thalassemia are shown in Figs. 2.1, 2.2, and 2.3.

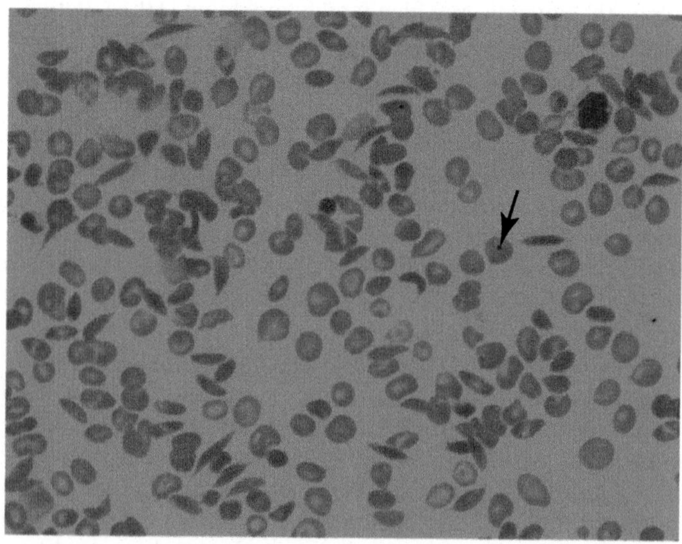

FIGURE 2.1 Blood film (×60) from patient with HbSS. There are numerous sickled cells. Polychromasia (blue/grey staining red cells) is prominent indicating an active bone marrow with increased young red cells in the circulation. There is also a Howell Jolly body (*arrow*) indicating hyposplenia

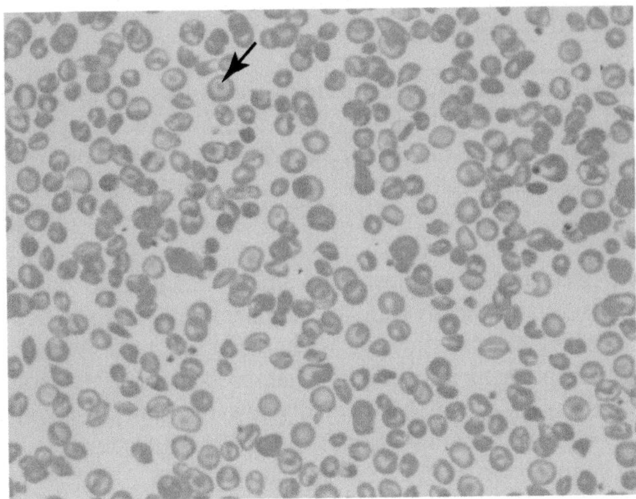

FIGURE 2.2 Blood film (×60) from patient with HbSC showing target cells (*arrow*) and contracted red cells which are smaller and densely staining. There are less sickled cells and less polychromasia than in HbSS

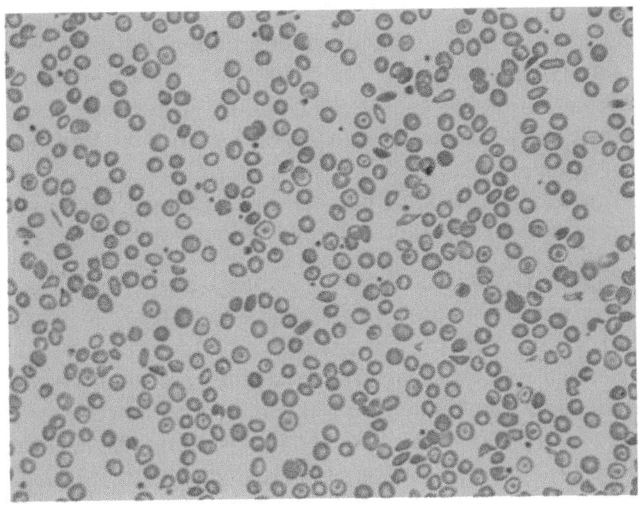

FIGURE 2.3 Blood film (×40) from child with HbS β° thalassemia, showing sickled cells, target cells and hypochromia (pale, poorly hemoglobinized cells)

Reticulocytes

The reticulocyte count is an indicator of the rate of red cell production in the bone marrow. The absolute reticulocyte count is more reliable than the percentage of reticulocytes, the latter being dependent on the overall red cell count. In steady state, the reticulocyte count is an important indicator of hemolytic rate and marrow response to hemolysis. During an acute vaso-occlusive or sequestration crisis, reticulocyte count is increased from steady state as the marrow responds to hemolytic stress. An aplastic crisis is characterized by a low reticulocyte response, due to temporary suppression of erythropoesis. Other causes of an unexpectedly low reticulocyte count in SCD include hematinic (iron, folate, B12) deficiency and marrow suppression from excessive hydroxyurea.

Analysis of Hemoglobin Type (Hemoglobinopathy Screen)

This has three main uses:

1. Diagnosis of SCD and differentiation between sickle genotypes.
2. Quantitation of sickle hemoglobin percentage during emergency exchange transfusion or chronic transfusion programme.
3. Quantitation of fetal hemoglobin percentage for assessment of prognosis and response to hydroxyurea therapy.

High performance liquid chromatography (HPLC) is the most common method of hemoglobin analysis in modern laboratories. Variant hemoglobins are identified by their shifted elution time from the ion exchange column compared with normal hemoglobin (HbA). The relative amounts of different hemoglobins can also be measured, and this is particularly useful for quantitation of hemoglobin A2 ($\alpha_2\gamma_2$) which is increased from <3.5 % to between 4 and 6 % in carriers of β thalassemia. HPLC is quick and reliable and can be automated to enable high throughput of samples. Typical chromatograms are shown in Fig. 2.4.

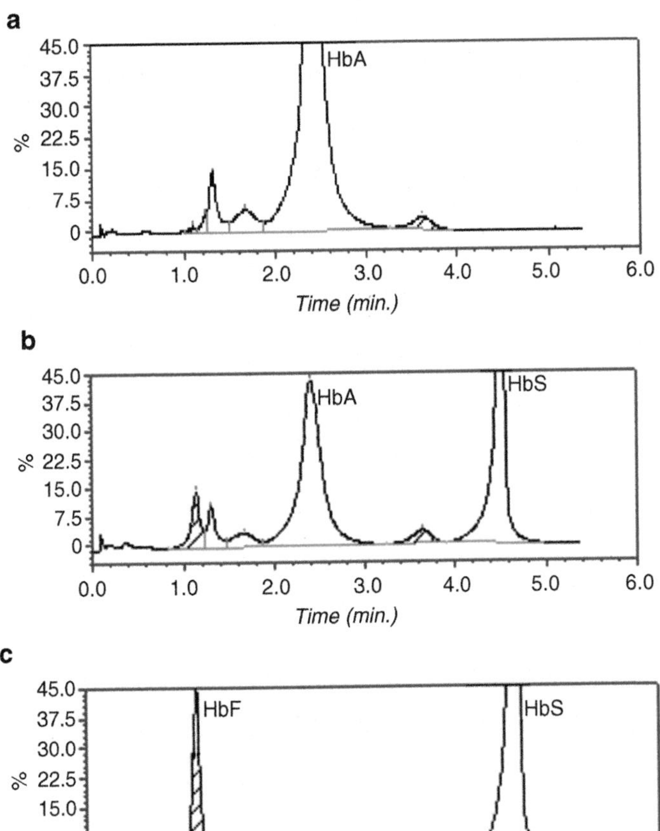

FIGURE 2.4 High pressure liquid chromatography HPLC traces (**a**) normal. (**b**) Carrier of HbS showing HbA (44 % of total hemoglobin) and HbS (40 %), (**c**) HbSS with high HbF (74 % HbS and 16 % HbF), (**d**) HbSC (44 % HbS and 44 % HbC), (**e**) HbS β^{+} thalassemia showing 16 % HbF, 15 % HbA, 5 % HbA2 and 53 % HbS. Note that the HPLC protocol is different in trace **e** compared to **a**–**d**, as shown by different retention times for the various hemoglobins

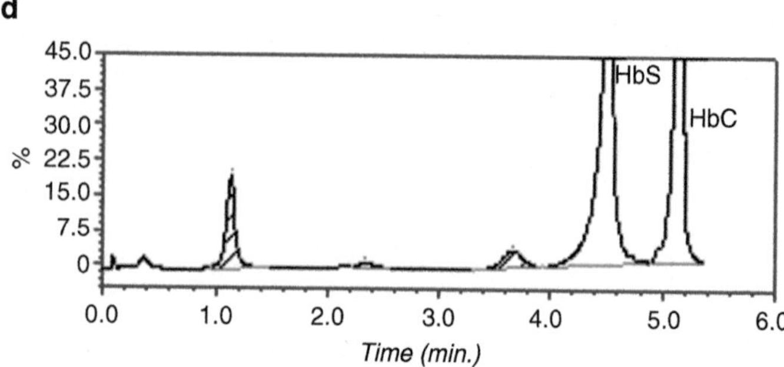

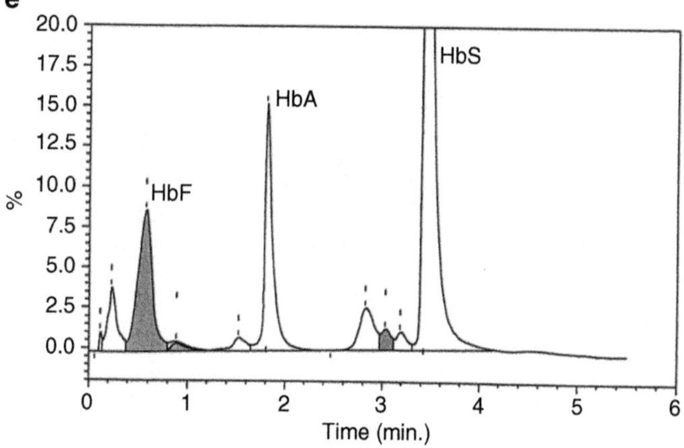

FIGURE 2.4 (continued)

HPLC by itself is not sufficient to confirm the identity of a variant hemoglobin and at least one further test is required. In the case of HbS, this is generally the sickle solubility test, which detects sickling of hemoglobin in solution with concentrated buffer treated with the reducing agent sodium metabisulphite (Fig. 2.5). If sickle hemoglobin is present at more than 10–15 % of total hemoglobin, the solution becomes cloudy. The test is specific for sickle hemoglobin, but does not differentiate between HbAS, HbSS and other compound heterozygotes of HbS.

Hemoglobin electrophoresis was the first method developed to demonstrate hemoglobin variants. It is more time

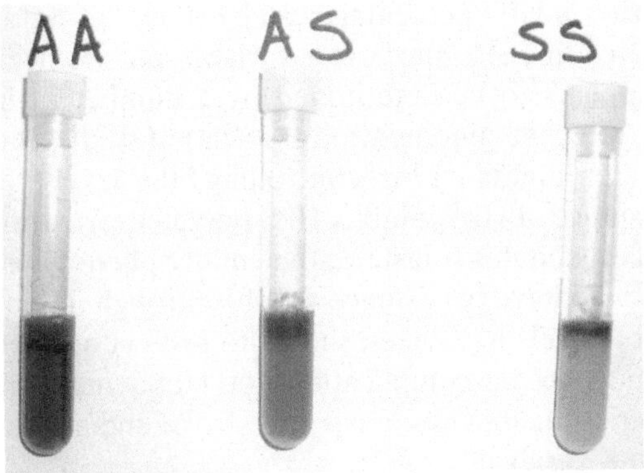

FIGURE 2.5 Sickle solubility test

consuming and labour intensive than HPLC, and in modern laboratories is now mainly used for confirming results obtained with HPLC. Laboratories with limited resources, particularly in low income countries, still use electrophoresis for diagnosis and carrier screening.

Alternative methodology is being introduced which identifies the variant directly, so that confirmatory testing is not required. These methods are DNA sequence analysis (which identifies the specific globin gene mutation), and Tandem Mass Spectrometry, which identifies the specific amino acid changes in the globin chain from a spectrogram produced from globin chain fragments generated by enzymatic digestion. These methods can potentially increase the speed and accuracy of analysis and may soon become routine methodology for diagnosis and screening.

Fetal Hemoglobin (HbF)

Fetal hemoglobin (HbF, $\alpha_2\gamma_2$) is the predominant hemoglobin produced during fetal development from 12 weeks up to term. Adult hemoglobin (HbA, $\alpha_2\beta_2$) predominates after the third month of life. In a normal individual, HbF is usually less than 1 % of total hemoglobin by 2 years of age but the rate of decrease in HbF percentage can be slower in children with SCD. After this age, there is a variable persistence of HbF which appears to be determined by a number of inherited elements. Recent genome wide association studies have identified the predominant loci controlling HbF levels.

Persistence of HbF inhibits HbS polymer formation within the red cell, and this translates to a milder phenotype in those patients who have persistence of HbF through into adult life. High HbF levels have been shown to protect against several acute and chronic complications of HbSS including acute painful crisis, acute chest crisis and stroke and are associated with better survival.

Bibliography

Ryan K et al. Significant hemoglobinopathies: guidelines for screening and diagnosis. Br J Haematol. 2010;149:35–49.

Chapter 3
Organization of Care

Introduction

In common with other long-term conditions, sickle cell disease presents a variety of clinical, psychological and social challenges for the patient and his/her carers. When organising services (Fig. 3.1), it is important to consider several particular features of the condition:

1. It is highly variable in clinical severity
2. The natural history entails an accumulation of long-term complications, punctuated by frequent, unpredictable episodes of acute illness
3. In England, other Northern European countries and North America, it is mainly restricted to ethnic minority groups, particularly black African and Caribbean populations.

The usual model for care requires a team of specialist medical and nursing practitioners interacting with a range of other professionals. The majority of care could be delivered from a community base, but in practice this has been difficult to achieve. Further studies to evaluate different methods of health care delivery are needed.

Hospital-based care is essential for management of acute complications, day care interventions such as transfusion and exchange transfusion, specialist clinic appointments and for laboratory and radiological investigations. Examples of care

J. Howard, P. Telfer, *Sickle Cell Disease in Clinical Practice*, In Clinical Practice, DOI 10.1007/978-1-4471-2473-3_3,

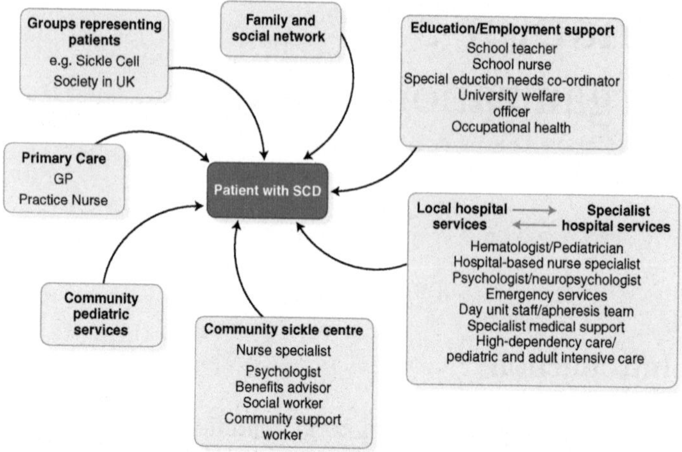

FIGURE 3.1 Components of the care network for a child or adult with SCD

that could be based either in the hospital or the community include routine out-patient appointments and annual reviews, monitoring of hydroxyurea and iron chelation therapy and management of some chronic complications, such as leg ulcers and chronic pain. Psychological support and social care, liaison with schools, employers, welfare benefit and housing officers are probably best delivered from a community setting.

The current model of care as described in UK national guidelines and supported by the National Hemoglobinopathy Screening Programme and Specialist Commissioning is based on a clinical network co-ordinated by a Specialist Center in a large hospital, which supports local hospital-based centers and community centers in their region. This model will hopefully encourage equitable, accessible and high quality care in low and high prevalence areas.

Specialist Centers

As well as providing specialist services the specialist center is responsible for annual review of all patients, management of complex acute and chronic complications, harmonization of treatment protocols and referral pathways, gathering and reporting of health outcome data, co-ordination of staff education, audit of on-going practice and for co-ordinating research including basic science and clinical trials.

Local Hospital Centers

In high prevalence areas, local centers may manage very large numbers of patients and have an established team of specialist doctors and nurses. In low prevalence areas, the numbers of patients may be very few and resources and skills correspondingly limited. In each case, the objectives of the local center should be the provision of routine care at a high standard, close to the patient's home, with good communication and agreed referral pathways to the specialist center. Routine care includes management of uncomplicated acute crises, administration of regular transfusions, and routine outpatient care.

Community Sickle Cell and Thalassemia Centers

In the 1970s and 1980s community-based sickle and thalassemia (SCAT) centers were established in high prevalence districts in London, Birmingham and Manchester. They were modeled on some of the practices developed by the comprehensive care centers in Jamaica and USA but were more community focused. The model which has developed in low prevalence areas is a single community base covering a larger region, or a more limited outreach service based in the local hospital. Implementation of antenatal and neonatal hemoglobinopathy screening is now an important activity in many of the SCAT centers, and is monitored through adherence to the standards of the national screening programme.

The pathway for neonatal screening starts with the reception of a positive neonatal screen result. Parents are then informed that they have affected offspring. Usually this requires several home visits during which the parents receive information about SCD and are offered various forms of support. Staff need to ensure that the infant is prescribed and adheres to penicillin prophylaxis, receives the relevant vaccinations and is referred to the local and specialist center for regular follow-up.

The pathway for antenatal screening starts with receiving results of the carrier mother, offering counselling and screening of the father, and organising prenatal diagnosis for at-risk pregnancies. In some areas these roles may be taken on by appropriately trained midwifery staff.

SCAT staff also have a key role in clinical, psychological and social support. Staff make visits to assess the home situation, and to anticipate difficulties in caring for an affected child. Continuing eduction about the condition is an important part of the role. Community based nurses are helpful in visiting schools to help ensure awareness and proper integration into normal school activities. They also provide a link between hospital and community, attending hospital outpatient clinics and visiting patients when they are admitted to hospital.

Primary Care

Although SCD specialists often try to take on the role of General Practitioner, this is a disservice to their patients, and obstructs integrated health care. Good communication, advice and education are key elements to ensure that the partnership works. The role of the GP includes routine primary health care and management of unrelated medical problems. GPs should be able to make an assessment of acute and chronic complications of SCD and arrange urgent or non-urgent specialist referrals as required. They are responsible for routine prescriptions of prophylactic antibiotics, folic acid, analgesic medications for use at home, and administration of vaccines (hepatitis B, Pneumovax®, influenza and additional catch up vaccinations if needed). They are also responsible for providing contraception and pregnancy advice, pre-conceptual counselling and suitable oral analgesia for acute painful episodes managed at home. Prescriptions of more specialized medications which need regular monitoring, such as hydroxyurea or iron chelating drugs, are usually arranged from the specialist clinic. However, shared care arrangements for hydroxyurea prescription and monitoring are also an option, provided that there is a clear protocol and good communication between the GP and the hospital specialist.

Emergency Care

The majority of severe acute complications of SCD are initially managed in the Emergency Departments (ED). It is important that ED nursing and medical staff have sufficient knowledge and experience in SCD management, and that the means of communication with the specialist team are clearly understood. Management in ED should be guided by a general treatment protocol covering acute pain management and the initial steps in managing other acute complications such as Acute Chest Syndrome (ACS) and priapism. All emergency medical and nursing staff should receive training about SCD management.

In-Patient Care

During an acute hospital admission, the patient may be managed by a specialist SCD team or by general pediatric/medical staff. Any medical or nursing staff looking after acutely unwell patients with SCD should have regular training updates to ensure adequate knowledge of the condition and familiarity with the treatment protocols. Hematologists and pediatricians in low prevalence areas may find themselves presented with patients in extremis and should be able to treat the acute emergencies of SCD, and to offer emergency exchange transfusion if required. In larger centers, acute hemoglobinopathy clinical nurse specialists are often a vital part of the specialist team.

Outpatient Care

Newly diagnosed infants should be seen within three months of birth and then regularly (at least six monthly). Older children and adults should have an annual specialist out-patient review. These out-patient appointments will often be multidisciplinary and include review by medical, nursing and psychology staff. They may have a 'one-stop' format, e.g. combining annual review with Transcranial Doppler scan. For more complex problems joint specialist clinics can be very successful and rewarding for the patient, family and health care staff. Large specialist centers have established speciality clinics in pediatric and adult services, providing a resource for patients within the wider clinical network. Examples include obstetrics, renal, endocrinology, orthopedics, urology, neurology, hepatology and chronic pain.

Psychology

Both clinical psychologists and health psychologists have an important role to play. The best results are obtained when the psychologist regularly participates in ward rounds, outpatient clinics and multidisciplinary meetings and becomes an integral part of the team. The role may include one-to-one support, cognitive behavioural therapy, acute interventions and support groups. Another important role is provision of neuropsychological assessment and support as part of the care of children with educational problems and cognitive difficulties.

Multidisciplinary Care and Other Agencies

Physiotherapisits, play specialists, dieticians, hospital school teachers, social workers and benefits officers all have an important role to play, and their contribution is greatly enhanced if they are part of a multi-disciplinary team. In this way they obtain a better understanding of the condition, become part of long-term care in the service and gain the confidence and acceptance of the patients and families.

User Groups and the Voluntary Sector

Most countries with a significant sickle cell population will have one or more national patient organizations and local groups. Some of these larger groups have had an important influence on national policy and help with patient advocacy and support. Examples include Sickle Cell Disease Association of America, Inc www.sicklecelldisease.org and the UK Sickle Cell Society (www.sicklecellsociety.org).

Bibliography

Standards for the linked Antenatal and Newborn Screening Programme. 2nd ed. 2011. www.Sct.screening.nhs.uk

Part II
Acute and Chronic Complications of Sickle Cell Disease

Chapter 4
Overview and General Principles

Management of Acute Complications

Most, but not all acute presentations are due to complications of sickle cell disease (SCD). Health care professionals who are unfamiliar with SCD sometimes fail to recognise a characteristic syndrome related to SCD and may attribute the symptoms and signs to a more familiar general medical diagnosis. This may result in incorrect management, with severe consequences. Conversely, in units where SCD is commonly seen, symptoms are assumed to be a 'sickle crisis' and insufficient consideration is given to alternative general medical conditions. This might happen in the situation of a young SCD child presenting with a febrile illness due to a viral infection, or an older patient with complications of diabetes or hypertension.

In this section we will describe the presentation, pathophysiology and management of complications of SCD. These are summarised in Table 4.1.

Patients, parents and carers are understandably anxious about falling ill and there is a common belief that children and young adults are likely to die from SCD. Explanation and education helps to empower patients to recognise and manage complications at home and understand when worrying symptoms are developing which need urgent medical attention. Some of these are listed in Table 4.2.

J. Howard, P. Telfer, *Sickle Cell Disease in Clinical Practice*, In Clinical Practice, DOI 10.1007/978-1-4471-2473-3_4,

TABLE 4.1 Complications of SCD

System	Acute complication	Chronic complication
Acute and chronic pain pathways	Acute painful crisis (APC)	Musculoskeletal pain
		Neuropathic pain
		Central sensitization syndromes
Musculoskeletal	Dactylitis	Avascular necrosis
	Acute bone infarction	Femoral head
	Osteomyelitis	Humeral head
		Vertebral bodies
		Chronic osteomyelitis
Cardiorespiratory	Acute chest syndrome (ACS)	Pulmonary hypertension (PHT)
		Asthma
		Chronic sickle lung syndrome
		Sleep disordered breathing
		Myocardial impairment

Brain	Acute ischemic stroke (AIS)	Silent cerebral ischemia (SCI)
	Transient ischemic attack (TIA)	Chronic ischemic damage with recurrent ischemic stroke
	Acute hemorrhagic stroke (AHS)	Vasculopathy
	Intracerebral hemorrhage (ICH)	Arterial stenosis
	Subarachnoid hemorrhage (SAH)	Arterial aneurysm
	Subdural haemorrhage (SDH)	Moyamoya
	Venous sinus thrombosis	Headache
	Posterior reversible encephalopathy syndrome (PRES)	Cognitive dysfunction
	Seizures	
	Infection	
	Bacterial meningitis	
	Viral meningitis	
	Cerebral abscess	
	Cerebral malaria	

(continued)

TABLE 4.1 (continued)

System	Acute complication	Chronic complication
Renal	Acute renal failure	Enuresis
	Hematuria	Proteinuria
	Urinary tract infection	Chronic renal failure
Urogenital	Priapism	Erectile dysfunction
Ophthalmological	Vitreous hemorrhage	Visual loss
	Retinal artery occlusion	
	Retinal detachment	
Spleen	Acute splenic sequestration (ASS)	Chronic splenomegaly
		Splenic dysfunction

Infection	Acute bacterial infection	Chronic osteomyelitis
	Meningitis	
	Osteomyelitis	
	Pneumonia	
	Septicemia	
	Urinary tract infection	
	Viral infection	
	Parvovirus B19 aplastic crisis	
	Transfusion transmitted viral infection (Hepatitis B, C, HIV)	
	Malaria	
	Falciparum, vivax, malariae, ovale	

(continued)

TABLE 4.1 (continued)

System	Acute complication	Chronic complication
Gastrointestinal	Abdominal sickle crisis (sometimes referred to as mesenteric crisis or girdle syndrome)	Pica (in children)
	Gallstone disease	Constipation
	Biliary colic	Chronic liver disease (sometimes referred to as sickle hepatopathy)
	Obstructive jaundice	
	Acute pancreatitis	
	Acute cholecystitis	
	Acute hepatic sequestration	
	Acute hepatic failure	
Dermatological		Chronic lower limb ulceration
Growth and endocrine		Growth impairment
		Delayed puberty
		Azospermia

TABLE 4.2 Indications for hospital review of sickle cell patients
Severe pain which does not settle with home analgesia
Chest pain and difficulty breathing
High fever and/or rigors
Pain associated with unusually severe headache
Severe lethargy or diminished level of consciousness
Priapism
Severe jaundice

There are a number of standard baseline investigations which are listed in Table 4.3.

Table 4.3 Routine blood tests for acute presentations with SCD

Investigation	Purpose	Comment
Full blood count	Routine for Acute painful crisis (APC) and other acute crises	Low hemoglobin compared to steady state –may be due to hemolysis, sequestration or concurrent aplastic crisis
		Raised white cell count – may indicate infection, but may also be seen in uncomplicated APC
		Raised platelet count – may be associated with severe painful episode.
		Low platelet count- may be spurious but is also seen in malaria, Acute Chest Syndrome (ACS) and hypersplenism
Reticulocytes	Investigation of low hemoglobin compared to steady state	Raised level indicates increased hemolysis or sequestration.
		Low level indicates aplastic crisis. Rarely due to hematinic deficiency, excessive hydroxyurea dosage or another hematological disorder.
Renal function	Routine for APC and other acute crises	Raised creatinine above steady state level – severe dehydration, sepsis (particularly pyelonephritis), severe acute sickling, non-steroidal anti-inflammatory drugs (NSAID's), diuretics, antibiotics, iron chelating agents, acute hemolytic transfusion reactions.

Liver function	Routine for APC and other acute crises	Raised bilirubin – increased hemolysis (acute sickling, transfusion reactions), acute hepatic complications (hepatic sequestration, obstructive jaundice), sepsis, drugs. Increased hepatitic enzymes (alanine transaminase, ALT and aspartate transaminase, AST) – hepatic complications (hepatic sequestration, hepatopathy), sepsis, drugs. Increased cholestatic enzymes (Alkaline phosphatase and gamma glutamyl transaminase) – cholestasis or biliary tract obstruction
C-reactive protein	Acute febrile illness	CRP may be elevated in steady state, and more so during any acute crisis. Sustained very high levels may indicate bacterial infection and may be useful in monitoring and management of certain infections (e.g. osteomyelitis)
Transfusion compatibility testing	If transfusion indicated	If there is no previous transfusion record, ABO group, extended red cell phenotype and antibody screen should be requested. Transfusion laboratory made aware of the diagnosis of SCD and of special blood requirements (See Chap. 18) For subsequent episodes, blood grouping, antibody screen and save serum should be requested.

Bibliography

Sickle cell disease in childhood. Standards and guidelines for clinical care. 2nd ed. 2010. www.sct.screening.nhs.uk.

Standards for the clinical care of adults with sickle cell disease in the UK. Sickle Cell Society. 2008. www.sicklecellsociety.

Chapter 5
Pain in Sickle Cell Disease

Acute Pain Crisis

Definition

The Acute Painful Crisis (APC) is an episode of pain, usually of abrupt onset, which in severe cases requires hospital treatment with opioid analgesia. Since there is no diagnostic test for APC, other potential causes of pain need to be excluded.

Etiology

APC is thought to be a clinical consequence of sickle hemoglobin-containing red blood cells becoming trapped in the microcirculation, leading sequentially to ischemia, infarction, reperfusion, and inflammation. Within the bone marrow, the result of this process is local tissue damage and increased intra-osseous pressure, together with the release of a variety of chemical mediators. These activate nociceptive neural pathways in the peripheral and central nervous system, leading to the perception of pain. Some features of APC, for instance the mechanism whereby trigger factors (temperature changes, infection, over-exertion, physical

J. Howard, P. Telfer, *Sickle Cell Disease in Clinical Practice*, In Clinical Practice, DOI 10.1007/978-1-4471-2473-3_5,

and psychological stress) lead to the onset of crisis, and the mechanisms whereby the site of pain changes and multiple sites of pain are recruited during the course of the episode, are poorly understood.

Incidence

APC is by far the commonest acute complication of SCD, but is highly variable in frequency. The majority of episodes are managed at home and usually go unrecorded. These mild episodes nevertheless result in significant morbidity, including exclusion from education, work and social activities as well as psychological maladaptation. Assessing frequency using a pain diary, or by careful systematic enquiry at routine out-patient clinic visits is important.

A recent American study showed that adults experienced pain on 50 % of days but only access health care services on 3 % of days. Another study found that patients have an average of 2.5 acute care encounters and 1.5 hospital admissions per year. Twenty-nine percent of patients do not seek acute care at all, whilst 16 % have 3 or more acute care encounters over 1 year.

The incidence of APC tends to increase during childhood and peak in adolescence and early adulthood, and in this age range is more common in males (Fig. 5.1). Pain crises become less frequent in patients over the age of 40.

UK Health Service Perspective

NHS hospital treatment episodes with a diagnosis of SCD doubled over the previous 10 years to about 25,000 per annum by 2009/10. On average, a patient will be admitted once per year, for 3–4 days. The majority of admissions are in London and occur most frequently in the age group 15–25 years. SCD is also the commonest reason for repeated readmissions to hospital within 28 days in London.

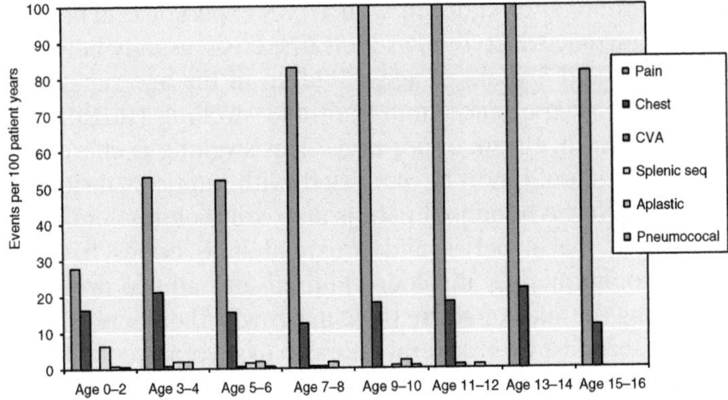

FIGURE 5.1 Age specific rates of acute painful crisis and other acute complications in the East London Newborn Cohort (data from HbSS children)

Presentation, Course and Complications

Typical precipitating factors include exposure to adverse weather conditions (particularly cold wind or rain) with inadequate clothing, over exertion, swimming in cold water, and psychological stress including family crises, school and university exams. APC can also accompany other acute complications, such as acute anemic episodes, infections, abdominal and respiratory crises, and may be a feature of some delayed transfusion reactions. Sometimes there is no apparent trigger. Patients are often able to recognise a prodrome of malaise, fatigue and gradual onset of pain. Pain may be intermittent and fluctuate in location, but usually there is a specific site or sites of maximum intensity. Ballas et al. have studied a large number of APC episodes and have described the evolution of pain and biomarkers in a four-stage scheme (1) prodromal (2) initial infarctive (3) established and (4) resolving (see http://asheducationbook.hematologylibrary.org/content/2007/1/97.full). Fever and increased inflammatory markers are typical of the later stages of a crisis, and the patient is often incorrectly diagnosed as suffering from infection.

About 50 % of children with HbSS experience hand and foot syndrome (dactylitis) as their first crisis, usually between 6 months and 3 years of age. Children in the age range 2–5 years often experience limb pain and swelling (thigh, shin, knee, forearm, elbow, upper arm). This swelling is characteristic, and should not be confused with septic arthritis or osteomyelitis. Abdominal pain is also common in childhood. The chest, back, pelvis and proximal limb bones become more common sites in older children and adults, probably reflecting the sites of active bone marrow in these age groups.

APC can last from several hours up to several weeks. More prolonged episodes are probably related to extensive bone infarction and a lengthy phase of inflammation and healing. In adults it is common for pain to persist after discharge from acute hospital care, and recurrences of acute pain requiring readmission to hospital are part of the typical course. These may be related to increased blood viscosity due to high levels of inflammatory mediators and to the adhesive properties of reticulocytes which increase as the bone marrow recovers.

One of the most important complications of APC is acute chest crisis (ACS). Monitoring for development of ACS with regular assessment of respiratory rate, oxygen saturation and daily examination of the chest is an essential part of the management of APC.

Diagnosis

There are no specific diagnostic tests for APC. This is a clinical diagnosis based on the patient's history, the similarity to previous episodes of APC, and exclusion of other possible causes of pain.

Assessment and Investigations

A proforma capturing the important points in the history and examination is shown in Appendix 1. The essential baseline observations should include pain score, sedation score, respiratory rate and oxygen saturation.

Essential laboratory and radiological examinations are shown in Table 4.3. Hemoglobin electrophoresis is not routinely required (HbS% does not change during APC).

Home Management

Patients and their families should be taught how to recognise and manage pain at home, but they should also be aware of the triggers for hospital attendance and medical review (see Table 4.2 in Chap. 4).

Hospital Management

The care pathway for APC needs to carefully planned and explained. Usually, the patient presents to the emergency department (ED), and from there is transferred to an acute care ward. In high prevalence areas, there is often a dedicated ward. Monitoring of pain score and vital signs, together with administration of analgesia continues seamlessly along the journey from ED to the medical ward. One of the roles of a sickle cell nurse specialist is to facilitate and co-ordinate this care pathway. Staff need to develop expertise in pain management, and should be able to identify signs of deterioration, and develop an understanding of the patient's perspective in order to provide sympathetic and responsive care. Training of medical and nursing staff is important and will influence outcomes, in terms of efficacy, safety and patient satisfaction with the care pathway.

Day Care management is a suitable alternative model of care for uncomplicated APC episodes. Patients can be assessed and treated rapidly by a specialized team of nurses and doctors. A limited number of boluses of strong opiate analgesia can be given, either by mouth or by injection. At the end of the day, the patient can be discharged home, provided no additional complications develop, and that there is a carer present to observe and support the patient at home. The patient can reattend the next day if necessary. Day Care management is generally preferred by patients, and can lead to substantial cost savings if hospital admissions are prevented. This care model works best with extended opening hours, since the majority of acute presentations occur outside of the working day.

Analgesia

Opioid analgesics are nearly always needed for management of moderate to severe pain. The history of previous exposure to opioid drugs is important, as opioid-naive patients are in general more sensitive to opioids than those who are have previously been exposed. A minority of patients, particularly adult, experience acute–on-chronic pain, and manage their symptoms with large and frequent doses of opioid analgesics in the community. These patients are tolerant of relatively high doses of opioids, and may attend hospital for additional analgesia on a frequent basis.

Morphine is generally considered the opioid of choice, however concerns have been raised about the high rate of adverse effects, and increased incidence of ACS. The analgesic effect and potential toxicity is enhanced by persistence of one of the drug metabolites, the 6-glucuronide conjugate. Alternative opioids used in the UK include diamorphine and oxycodone.

British Committee for Standards in Haematology (BCSH), and National Institute for Clinical Excellence (NICE) guidelines recommend analgesia is given within 30 min of arrival in the ED. The intravenous route is the quickest method of obtaining therapeutic benefit, but in practice, delays often occur in prescribing, drawing up, checking and obtaining intravenous access. Alternative means of administering rapid acting opioid analgesia can be considered.

For continued pain management the commonest regime used in the UK is opioid injection given as repeated bolus. This regime does not allow for smooth, sustained analgesia, and demands intensive input from nursing staff. The patient controlled analgesia (PCA) device is better, since it gives the patient more control over treatment, and circumvents the need for repeated injections administered by nursing staff

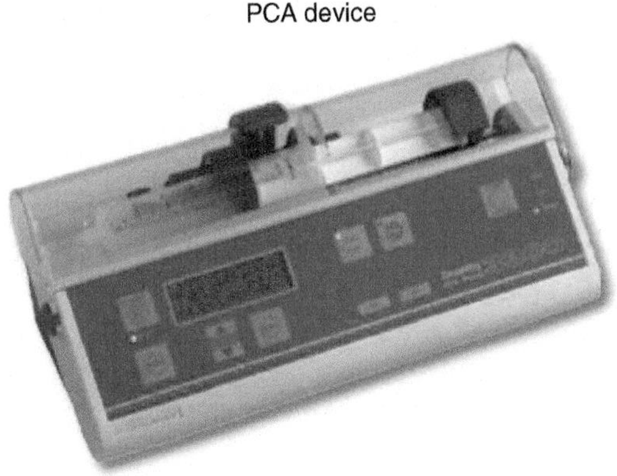

FIGURE 5.2 Patient controlled analgesia (PCA) device

(Fig. 5.2). Patients on PCAs require regular observation, particularly if having a continuous background infusion. There is a potential of unnecessarily high exposure to injected opiates and this may prolong hospital admission, and restrict mobilization. In children, an oral regimen consisting of short-acting morphine (Oramorph®) and long-acting morphine (Morphine Sulphate Tablet) for background analgesia has been shown to be as effective as intravenous morphine via PCA. Examples of analgesia protocols are shown in Appendix 2.

Monitoring

Opioid drugs are potentially toxic and inappropriate dosing can result in excess morbidity and mortality, particularly from respiratory suppression and excessive sedation. Frequent monitoring of vital observations including respiratory rate and sedation score are mandatory. We recommend hourly monitoring of respiratory rate, sedation score and oxygen saturation for the first 6 h after admission, and thereafter at least 4 h. For assessment of pain score in children, we use a scoring system from 0 to 3 which combines patients perception (with a faces score) and staff perception. For adults, we prefer a 0–10 visual analogue scale (Appendix 3).

Fluids

In most patients oral fluids can be used, and intravenous fluids restricted to those with clinical signs of dehydration, vomiting, diarrhoea or abdominal crises who should be nil by mouth. If intravenous fluids are required these can be given at maintenance rate. There is no evidence that 'hyper-hydration' is of benefit.

Additional Measures

Additional Analgesia

Paracetamol and non-steroidal anti-inflammatory agents (NSAIDs) can be prescribed, initially on a regular basis. These may help to limit opioid exposure. Excessive and prolonged dosing with NSAIDs can contribute to renal impairment and fluid retention in severe crises.

Management of Opioid Adverse Effects

Laxatives, antiemetics and antipruritics should be prescribed. The opioid antagonist naloxone is helpful for severe opioid adverse effects (respiratory depression, sedation, urinary retention).

Nitrous oxide (Entonox)

This is very helpful in the ambulance and on arrival in hospital, but should not be used over a prolonged period of time during admission with APC because of the risk of megaloblastic anemia and neuropathy.

Oxygen

Inhaled oxygen should be given if pulse oximetry shows that oxygen saturations are below the patient's known baseline or <95 % on air.

Blood Transfusion

This is not routinely indicated for the management of acute painful crisis, but can be considered where the hemoglobin has fallen significantly (<20 g/l below baseline), or where other complications develop.

Incentive Spirometry (Fig. 5.3)

This is recommended in older children and adults with chest pain, back pain, or chest infection. Performed regularly every two hours, it has been shown to decrease the risk of ACS and atelectasis.

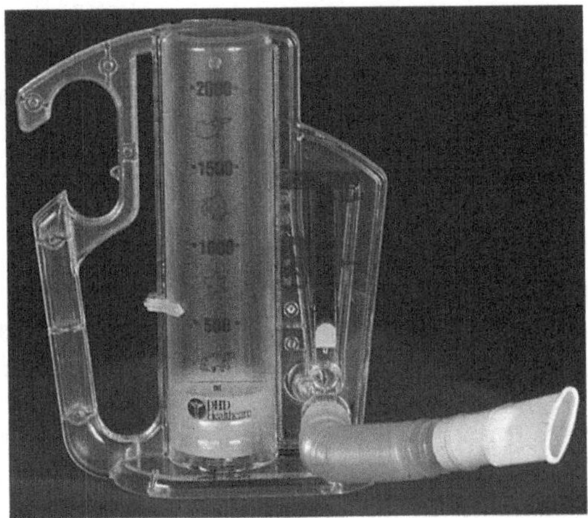

FIGURE 5.3 Incentive spirometer. This is used to encourage deep inspiration and lung expansion in children and adults with chest or high back pain, and after surgery

Antibiotics

Fever is a feature of APC, and antibiotics should not be prescribed for low grade fever in the context of APC without other evidence of infection. Of course, if there is a persistant fever or other features of infection (e.g. urinary or chest symptoms) appropriate antibiotics should be prescribed after blood or urine cultures have been taken.

Long-Term Management and Prevention of APC

APC is a distressing, disruptive and often unpredictable feature of the disease that has significant negative impact on quality of life and daily function. There are two complementary approaches to long-term management.

Self-Education and Psychological Support

This includes developing self-awareness about the effects of the disease, an understanding of what tends to trigger APC, and how to minimise the exposure to these trigger factors. In addition patients need to develop a personal method for dealing with APC when it occurs, how to distract, relax, avoid catastrophizing and minimize psychological stress. Courses of cognitive behavioural therapy may be helpful.

Medical Interventions to Reduce Frequency and Severity of APC

There are three therapeutic options which have been shown to be effective: Hydroxyurea, regular transfusion and bone marrow transplantation. These will be covered in Chap. 18.

Dactylitis

Dactylitis (Hand and foot syndrome) is often the first acute complication seen in a child with HbSS, and should be easily recognisable by an informed parent or GP. It is thought to be a variant of the acute painful crisis affecting the small bones of the hands and feet, parts of the skeleton that seem particularly vulnerable in young children perhaps because they are most exposed to cold.

In our cohort, dactylitis occurred in about 40 % of HbSS infants by the age of 2 years and was not common after the age of 5. It is unusual to see dactylitis in infants with milder sickle genotypes such as HbSC.

The infant is irritable and the affected hand or foot is puffy and uncomfortable to touch. Sometimes an individual digit is involved. Uncomplicated episodes resolve after a few days, and are generally easy to manage with increased oral fluids, paracetamol and a non-steroidal anti-inflammatory agent (ibuprofen for an infant). Dactylitis can be a feature of a more complex crisis and a small minority of children get frequent and distressing episodes from an early age. These children tend to have frequent painful crises and recurrent acute chest syndrome when they get older.

Chronic damage to the growth plates has been described resulting in shortened digits, but we have not observed this in our patients.

Chronic Pain

Definition

Chronic pain is a general term applied to long-lasting pain (persisting for more than 3 months). This includes a variety of different types of pain whose etiologies are still incompletely understood. In the case of SCD, chronic pain needs to be differentiated from a prolonged severe acute crisis or series of crises. These are expected to resolve eventually without long-term persistence of pain.

It is helpful to keep in mind the following categories when assessing chronic pain in SCD.

- Central Sensitization Syndromes – CSS (See etiology and physiology below)
- Hyperalgesia: Exaggerated pain response to normally mild stimuli. Associated with CSS and excessive opioid usage.
- Allodynia: Pain response to non-noxious stimuli. Also a feature of CSS and excessive opioid usage.
- Neuropathic pain: Pain caused by peripheral nerve or nerve root damage. In SCD this has been described involving spinal nerve roots, lingual nerve etc.
- Arthritic pain: Related to bone and joint damage from long-term effects of SCD. An example of this is avascular necrosis of the femoral and humeral head and of the vertebral bones.

Etiology and Pathogenesis

Chronic sickle pain is poorly understood. Conditions seen in general practice and chronic pain clinics (e.g. fibromyalgia, chronic headache, temporo-mandibular dysfunction) are a useful paradigm and are sometimes referred to as Central Sensitivity Syndromes (CSS). In these there is a general increased sensitivity to painful and non-painful stimuli and to other sensory inputs, such as loud noise. This is reflected in increased brain activity in areas associated with pain perception and emotional response to pain, notably the insula. Twin studies suggest a genetic predisposition. Central sensitivity appears to be precipitated and reinforced by repeated painful and stressful stimuli, and may be mediated by an enhanced transmission and reduced inhibition of nociceptive neural impulses at the level of the spinal cord, mid brain and cortex.

In SCD, long-term nociceptive inputs from acute vaso-occlusion, enhanced by psychological stress and a genetic predisposition, might result in widespread, higher intensity pain and pain of altered character. This alteration of the pain modulating pathways is difficult to reverse, and adversely affected by chronic use of opioid drugs.

Incidence

The definition and diagnostic criteria need to be better defined in order to describe the epidemiology. Pooled data from several studies suggest that as many as 50 % of patients may be suffering chronic pain, and some are experiencing severe symptoms every day. It is more common in adults than children, and perhaps in developed countries more than in Africa and the Caribbean. This may be related to the importance of opioid drugs in the etiology and the relatively restricted use of opioids in some countries where SCD is highly prevalent may lead to decreased levels of chronic pain.

Clinical Presentation

The typical features are of disabling, severe pain, which is not clearly localized, often described as 'all over body pain'. Some patients describe pain in the joints, lower extremities or back. Pain may vary in severity from day to day, but during bad spells, pain is constant, restricts activities and impacts significantly on working, family and social life. It also disrupts the normal sleep pattern. The pain often has typical features of hyperalgesia and/or allodynia. Characteristically, it is inadequately relieved by conventional analgesics, including opioids. Treatments directed against SCD, such as hydroxyurea or blood transfusion, are also not effective, and even after successful stem cell transplantation, pain may take many months to resolve. Psychological abnormalities suggestive of depression are common, and some patients have a history of high opioid use, despite not always being linked with frequent acute painful crisis.

Diagnosis

This is complicated by the overlap with acute painful crises. A pattern of unremitting pain, without the characteristic episodic nature of recurrent acute crises, and pain of a more generalized nature with hyperalgesia and allodynia should raise the possibility of chronic pain. Additional features include lack of response to opioid and other analgesics, and poor response to hydroxyurea or blood transfusions.

Pain associated with avascular necrosis of the hip or shoulder is described in Chapter 9. Chronic back pain is also common, and may be associated with a spectrum of vertebral and disc abnormalities on MRI, although there is often a dissociation between the severity of pain and MR findings. There is some evidence that Vitamin D deficiency may cause chronic musculoskeletal pain. Vitamin D deficiency is common in both children and adults with SCD, therefore we recommend levels should be checked in patients with chronic pain and deficiency treated promptly.

Management and Prevention

Managing chronic pain is challenging, and there are very few studies to guide therapy in SCD. The first step is to differentiate prolonged acute painful crisis and other causes of pain which require specific treatments (e.g. surgical treatment for avascular necrosis). We strongly recommend a multidisciplinary team approach involving a chronic pain specialist. General guidelines for managing chronic pain (e.g. British Pain Association, http://www.britishpainsociety.org/book_opioid_main.pdf), emphasizing acceptance, lifestyle change, psychological input (e.g. cognitive behavioural therapy, peer support groups) and graduated exercise programmes supervized by a physiotherapist may be beneficial. Some patients have found chronic pain management programmes helpful. Vitamin D supplementation should be considered in patients who are Vitamin D deficient.

Patients may benefit from medication to treat neuropathic pain (e.g. amitryptiline, gabapentin). In general, opioids are not recommended for managing chronic pain, and may exacerbate symptoms, however, in practice it may be difficult to wean patients who have used opioids for many years for acute painful crisis management.

Bibliography

Brousseau DC, Owens PL, Mosso AL, et al. Acute care utilization and rehospitalization for sickle cell disease. JAMA. 2010;303(13):1288–94.

Rees DC, et al. Guideline for the management of acute painful crisis in sickle cell disease. Br J Haematol. 2003;120:744–52.

Scottish Intercollegiate Guidelines Network. Management of chronic pain. Guideline no 136, Dec 2013. www.sign.ac.uk/guidelines/fulltext/136/.

Smith WR, Pemberthy LT, Bovbjerg VE, et al. Daily assessment of pain in adults with sickle cell disease. Ann Intern Med. 2008;148:92–101.

Chapter 6
Respiratory and Cardiac Complications

Acute Chest Syndrome

Definition

Acute chest syndrome (ACS) is a potentially life-threatening acute respiratory illness, often preceded by an acute painful crisis. It is characterized by fever, pleuritic chest pain, inspiratory crepitations on auscultation of the chest, and is accompanied by a new infiltrate on chest X-ray (CXR). The broadest definition is simply the presence of respiratory signs and symptoms and a new infiltrate on CXR. It is specific to sickle cell disease (SCD) and general physicians who are not familiar with SCD may misdiagnose ACS as pneumonia, pulmonary edema or adult respiratory distress syndrome and institute inappropriate treatment.

Etiology and Pathophysiology

A variety of insults can precipitate intrapulmonary vaso-occlusion, progressive hypoxemia and lung damage. An infective agent is sometimes identified, more often in children than adults. The most common infections diagnosed are *Chlamydia pneumoniae*, *Mycoplasma pneumoniae* and viruses causing pneumonia, including respiratory syncytial

J. Howard, P. Telfer, *Sickle Cell Disease in Clinical Practice*, In Clinical Practice, DOI 10.1007/978-1-4471-2473-3_6,

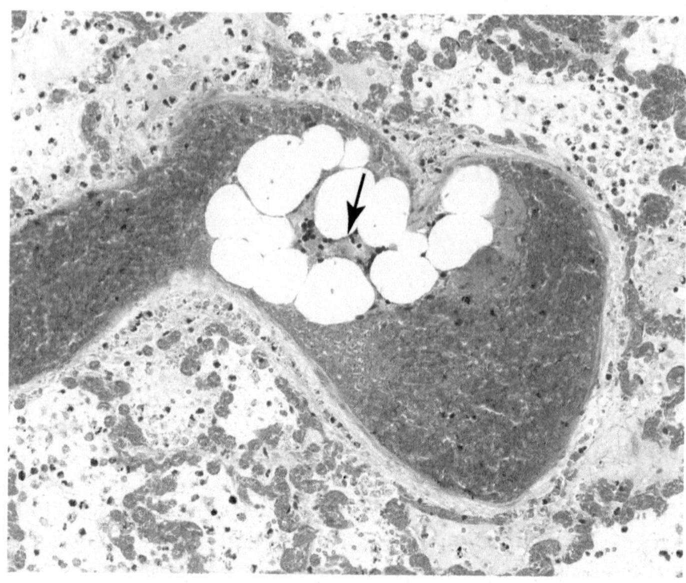

FIGURE 6.1 Post mortem histopathology section of lung from a patient with HbSS and acute chest syndrome. There is a prominent pulmonary vessel containing sickled red cells and marrow fat embolism (*arrow*)

virus. Bronchoscopic investigation has demonstrated fat laden macrophages in the airways, supporting the suggestion that acute fat embolism is important in the pathophysiology (Fig. 6.1). It is suggested that infarction of bone marrow during a severe acute painful crisis leads to necrosis and release of fat emboli which can lodge in the pulmonary vasculature. This provokes an acute inflammatory reaction with activation of the pulmonary endothelium leading to adhesion of leucocytes and sickled red cells. The result is a cycle of further hypoxia, sickling and vaso-occlusion. The mechanisms involved in vaso-occlusion, including hypoxia-reperfusion injury, free radical formation and activation of the coagulation proteins and platelets are likely to be involved in driving the process (see Fig. 1.4). Hypoventilation due to excessive pain during respiration, or opioid-induced respiratory suppression can exacerbate the situation further. The consequence of this cycle of insults can be appreciated from

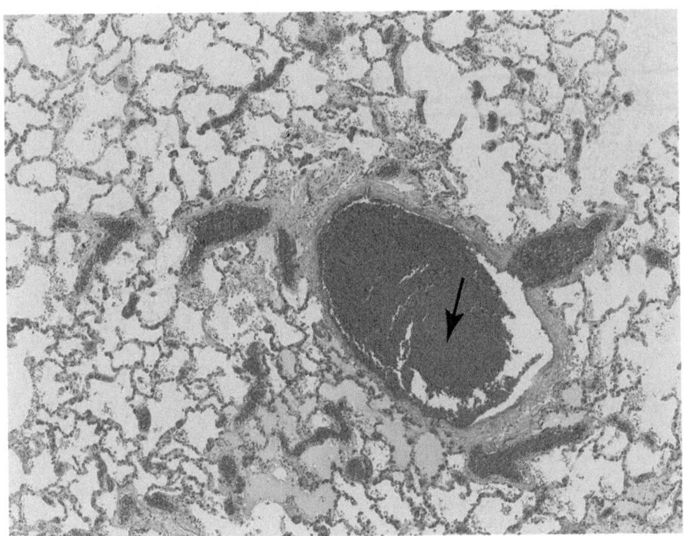

FIGURE 6.2 Histopathology of acute chest syndrome showing vessels congested with sickled red cells and thrombus (*arrow*)

post-mortem histology of patients who have died during a severe ACS episode. There is engorgement and occlusion of the pulmonary vasculature with sickled red cells, and sometimes accompanying widespread thrombotic occlusion (Figs. 6.2 and 6.3).

Risk Factors

These include high steady state hemoglobin and WBC, low HbF, a past history of ACS and of asthma.

Incidence

Incidence rates have reduced with increasing use of hydroxyurea in children and adults. Rates in the pre-hydroxyurea era were higher in young children, and in HbSS. In the East London Cohort, the overall rate in childhood for HbSS was 17 per 100 patient years and for HbSC 4 per 100 patient years.

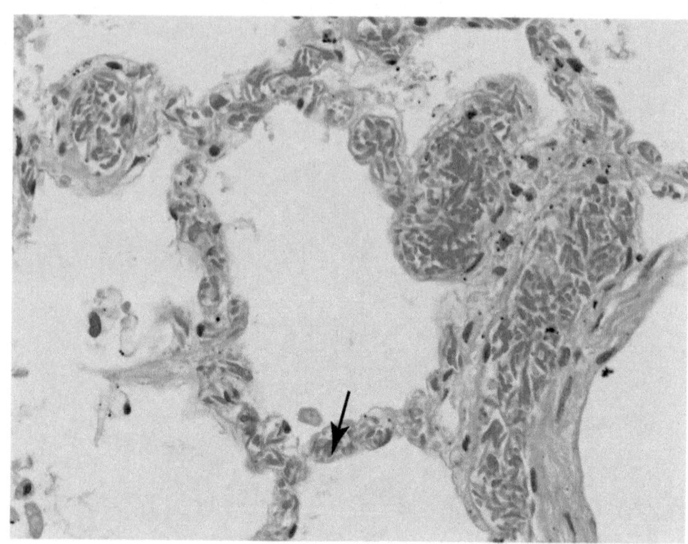

FIGURE 6.3 Histopathology of acute chest syndrome (high power) showing small blood vessels congested with sickled red cells surrounding alveolar spaces (*arrow*)

In the Co-operative Study of Sickle Cell Disease in North America (CSSD) the incidence in patients over 20 years of age was 8.7/100 person years. ACS is the second most common cause of admission to hospital after acute pain.

Clinical Presentation

Sometimes patients present with clinical features of ACS in the Emergency Department, but more commonly ACS is preceded by a severe painful crisis, and respiratory symptoms develop 24–72 h after the onset of pain, with evolving chest pain, together with fever and falling oxygen saturation on pulse oximetry. Regular monitoring of vital signs (in particular oxygen saturation) and chest examination are therefore essential during admission for painful crisis. The most common respiratory symptoms are cough, chest pain and shortness of breath. The chest pain may be felt in the ribs, sternum, or deeper within the chest, and restricts respiration. Wheezing and hemoptysis may also occur.

Low oxygen saturations (O_2 saturations <94 % or a fall of 3 % or more from baseline) is common, and a diagnosis of ACS should be considered in any hypoxic patients with SCD. On examination fever, tachypnoea (and intercostal recession in children), tachycardia and wheeze may be apparent. Chest examination is often abnormal, typically with inspiratory crepitations evolving into reduced breath sounds and signs of consolidation (bronchial breathing, reduced air entry, dullness to percussion) at the lung bases, either unilaterally or bilaterally. Although ACS is more common in HbSS, it can occur with similar severity in all genotypes and diagnosis and management are the same irrespective of genotype.

Clinical Course

The severity is very variable, ranging from a mild illness to a severe life threatening condition. In young children, the picture may resemble a lobar pneumonia, and chest pain is not so prominent, however, we frequently see a severe, rapidly progressive course in young children as well. ACS can progress rapidly to respiratory failure and a minority of patients will need mechanical ventilation. There is a risk of associated neurological complications including acute ischaemic stroke (AIS) and posterior reversible encephalopathy syndrome (PRES) and even without other complications, hospital admission is likely to be prolonged. ACS is a common cause of premature mortality in SCD and is a common cause of death in patients with SCD in the UK.

Differential Diagnosis

Other conditions to consider include pneumonia, pulmonary embolism, fluid overload and atelectasis with hypoventilation due to excessive pain or overdose of opioid analgesics.

Investigations

The investigations in Table 4.3 should always be requested. A fall in hemoglobin from steady state is almost universal, and is associated with markers of increased hemolysis. A low platelet count may be a marker of acute fat embolism and indicates that the course is likely to be more severe. Renal function may deteriorate, particularly in older patients with underlying chronic renal damage. CRP is not particularly helpful in distinguishing infection from acute vaso-occlusion, as it tends to be markedly raised during the course of ACS whatever the etiology. Additional essential investigations are listed in Table 6.1

TABLE 6.1 Additional investigations for ACS

Investigation	Purpose	Comments
Chest X-Ray	Location and extent of infiltration. Identification of pleural effusion, atelectasis, pulmonary edema.	May be normal early in ACS. The usual progression is from unilateral or bilateral basal opacification to involvement of multiple lung segments, air bronchograms, sometimes with pleural effusions (Fig. 6.4).
Arterial blood gas (on room air)	To assess gas transfer and acid-base balance	Should be done on air. Hypoxemia is very common. Decreasing pO_2 and increasing pCO_2 are indications for intensification of respiratory support and for exchange transfusion.

TABLE 6.1 (Continued)

Investigation	Purpose	Comments
Microbiological investigations	All cases of ACS	It is good practice to request bacterial culture of blood and sputum, PCR of nasopharyngeal aspirate, serology for atypical pneumonia, acute and convalescent samples for *Mycoplasma*, *Chlamydia*, *Legionella*, and urinary pneumococcal antigen.

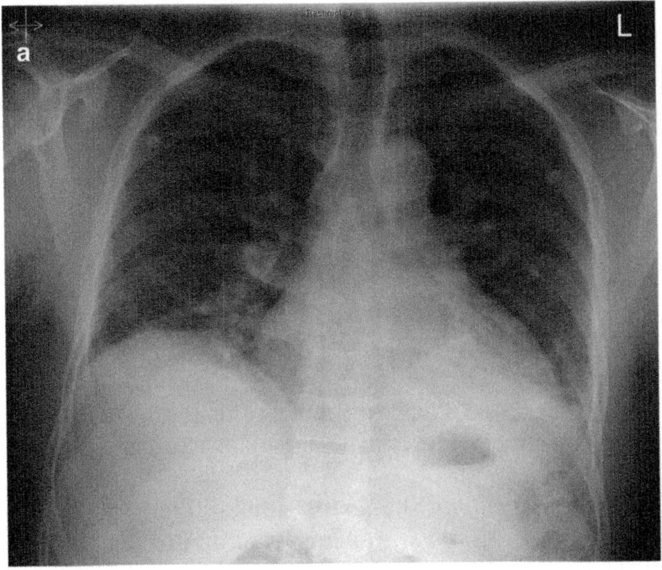

FIGURE 6.4 Chest X-rays of patient with acute chest syndrome. (**a**) Day 1, (**b**) Day 2, showing rapid progression of consolidation

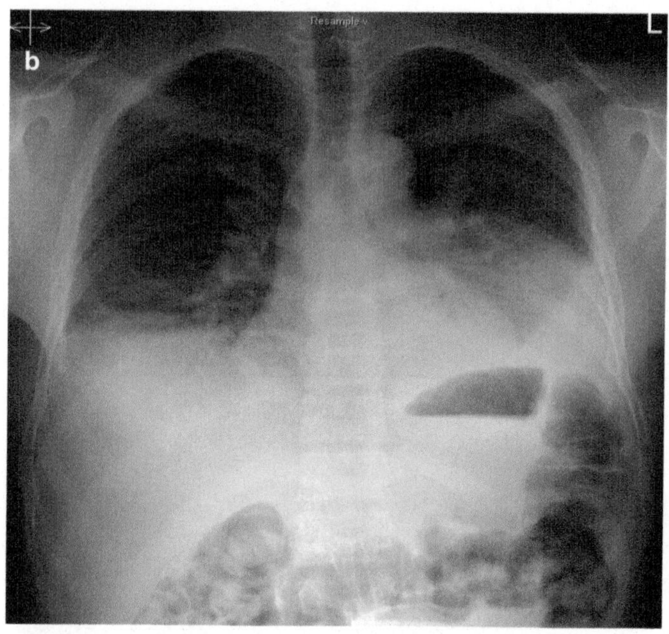

FIGURE 6.4 (Continued)

Management

ACS is a medical emergency, requiring early involvement of specialist hematology or pediatric hematology and critical care teams. A suggested management algorithm is shown in Fig. 6.5.

Oxygen should be given to maintain oxygen saturations >95 %.

Intravenous fluids should be administered to maintain adequate hydration, but it is important not to over-hydrate, particularly in the case of children. Fluid overload is a risk factor for posterior reversible encephalopathy syndrome (PRES) and may precipitate pulmonary edema in older patients with impaired renal function. Usually, replacement of daily fluid requirements is sufficient.

Analgesia is very important to control chest pain and permit adequate ventilation, but opioids must be used carefully to avoid over-sedation and respiratory suppression. Frequent

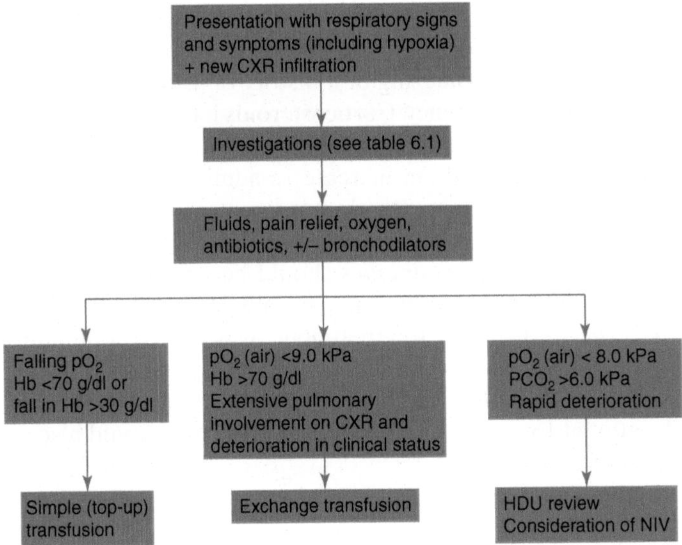

FIGURE 6.5 Algorithm for management of acute chest syndrome. *HDU* High dependency unit, *NIV* Non-invasive ventilation

monitoring of pain score, sedation score and respiratory rate is essential. One of the authors has found that intravenous fentanyl given by PCA is useful in this situation. Fentanyl is a potent synthetic opioid with a shorter half-life than morphine. Titration of opioid dose against pain is easier and there is less risk of opioid accumulation and overdosage.

Respiratory support and physiotherapy. There is evidence from a randomized clinical trial that incentive spirometry reduces the risk of ACS in children with chest pain. It is also useful as an adjunct to physiotherapy for ACS. In more severe cases, positive expiratory pressure devices (PEP) can be very helpful. These inputs help to optimize inspiratory effort and avoid atelectasis. Thick airway secretions often build up during the course of ACS, and are only expectorated as the condition resolves. Often they have a striking bright yellow colour due to bilirubin from breakdown of red cells in the lungs. These secretions can cause blockage or airways resulting in segmental collapse and further deterioration in respiratory state. Sedation and mechanical ventilation may be needed and early advice should be sought from the HDU or ITU teams.

Bronchodilators There is no clear evidence showing benefit of bronchodilators, but we recommend their use in patients with evidence of wheezing or a history of asthma in order to optimise airway patency. Corticosteroids have been shown to decrease the length of hospitalization with ACS, but have been associated with an increase re-admission rate because of rebound sickle pain. We do not use steroids routinely for ACS management.

Broad spectrum antibiotics should be prescribed at least until blood and sputum samples are shown to be negative. The local policy for treatment of a severe community acquired pneumonia should be followed, and this should include a macrolide antibiotic to cover atypical organisms. Treatment for the H1N1 subtype of influenza should also be considered.

Transfusion (See Chap. 18)

Blood transfusion can be lifesaving in severe ACS. Stabilization or improvement in respiratory status is often rapid, and it is important to avoid delay once the decision has been made to transfuse. The therapeutic effect is believed to be due to improved oxygen carriage, reduced sickling and relief of vaso-occlusion through dilution of sickled red cells in the microcirculation.

The decisions of when to transfuse, and whether to use simple or exchange transfusion can be difficult. They require clinical experience and are guided by an assessment of the clinical status and the risk of deterioration in respiratory function.

An initial simple transfusion is needed prior to exchange transfusion if the Hb has dropped to below 70 g/l. Simple transfusion can also be considered in a milder case of ACS, to prevent deterioration. If hemoglobin level permits (<80 g/l), we recommend transfusion of 10–20 ml/kg red cell concentrate. We have used this approach successfully on many occasions in both children and adults.

Exchange transfusion is indicated when there is a rapidly deteriorating clinical picture, with progressive chest signs, and worsening hypoxemia. An oxygen level of <9.0 kPa is sometimes used as an indication for transfusion but in patients who have a rapidly deteriorating clinical picture, transfusion should not be delayed if there is a lesser degree of hypoxia. Exchange transfusion can be performed either by a manual or automated approach. The objective is to maintain haemoglobin level between 80 and 110 g/l and to reduce HbS%. It is very important to avoid over-transfusion (Hb >110 g/l). In this situation, higher haemoglobin levels will increase blood viscosity, decrease the efficiency of tissue oxygen delivery, and may increase the risk of acute neurological events.

Chronic Sequelae

Pulmonary fibrosis, worsened lung function and chronic sickle lung disease have been described, however, these are not the inevitable consequence of episodes of ACS. Long-term out-patient monitoring of pulmonary status is particularly important in patients with a history of recurrent ACS.

Prevention

Hydroxyurea decreases the incidence and severity of ACS and is indicated in patients who have recurrent ACS or a single life-threatening episode. Long-term transfusion therapy is also very effective in preventing ACS and should be considered in patients who do not have a satisfactory response to hydroxyurea.

Pulmonary Hypertension

Increased pressure on the right side of the heart has become recognized as an important cause of chronic morbidity and mortality in SCD. There is still controversy about the diagnosis, pathophysiology, clinical significance, and management of

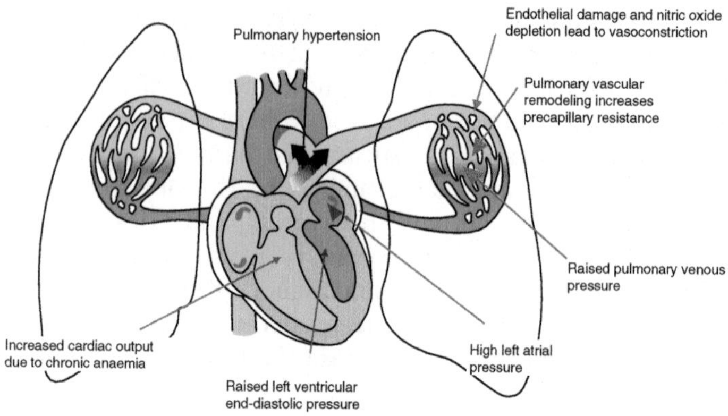

FIGURE 6.6 Cardio-pulmonary abnormalities which contribute to pulmonary hypertension in SCD

pulmonary hypertension (PHT), and for those who are not specialists in cardiopulmonary medicine, PHT is a confusing area.

Definition

PHT is defined as a resting mean pulmonary artery pressure (mPAP) of ≥25 mmHg directly measured at cardiac catheterization. The cardio-pulmonary circulation abnormalities giving rise to PHT are shown in Fig. 6.6 and Table 6.2. These may arise if pulmonary vascular resistance is increased, with or without an increase in cardiac output (precapillary PHT). Alternatively, or concurrently, there may be increased pressure on the left side of the heart e.g. from stiff left ventricle or mitral valve stenosis (postcapillary PHT). Back pressure due to a stiff left ventricle needs to be excluded by confirming a normal pulmonary artery wedge pressure during cardiac catheterization. Normally, patients with SCD have increased cardiac output and decreased blood viscosity as a result of anemia, and pulmonary vascular resistance is decreased compared to non-SCD controls. Patients with SCD may show features of precapillary or postcapillary PHT and some patients will have a raised mPAP with both a

TABLE 6.2 Pulmonary vascular measurements at cardiac catheterization in different categories of PHT

	Precapillary PHT	Postcapillary PHT	PHT with features of precapillary and postcapillary PHT
Mean pulmonary arterial pressure (mPAP)	≥25 mmHg	≥25 mmHg	≥25 mmHg
Pulmonary arterial wedge pressure (PAWP)	≤15 mmHg	>15 mmHg	>15 mmHg
Pulmonary vascular resistance	≥160 dyn·s·cm[5]	<160 dyn·s·cm[5]	≥160 dyn·s·cm[5]

raised pulmonary vascular resistance and an increased pulmonary arterial wedge pressure.

Elevated systolic pulmonary artery pressure has been shown to correlate with echocardiography measurements of tricuspid regurgitation velocity (TRV) and a raised TRV is associated with increased mortality in adults. At first, when this finding was published, a raised TRV was taken as a surrogate marker for PHT, however, it is becoming clear that not all patients with a raised TRV have PHT when assessed at cardiac catheterization, and that some have features of precapillary PAH, some of postcapillary PAH and some have features of both. The term 'pulmonary hypertension' should only refer to patients diagnosed by cardiac catheterization, not to those with a raised TRV alone.

Incidence

Up to 30 % of adult patient with HbSS have a raised TRV (>2.5 m/s) measured at echocardiography. In a large French study where diagnosis was confirmed by cardiac catheterization, the prevalence of PHT was 6 %, of whom around half had precapillary, and half postcapillary PHT. PHT and raised TRV are more common in patients with HbSS than other genotypes and the prevalence increases with age.

Pathophysiology

Both pulmonary vasoconstriction and endothelial dysfunction are thought to be involved. A proposed mechanism whereby chronic intravascular hemolysis leads to release of free hemoglobin and arginase which deplete and deregulates nitric oxide is described in Chap. 1. The process is also

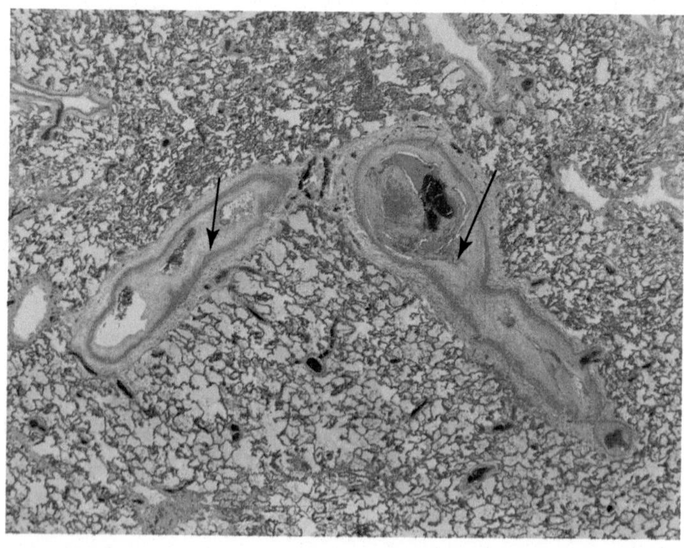

FIGURE 6.7 Post-mortem histology from the lung of an adult patient with HbSS and pulmonary hypertension showing arterial wall thickening and almost complete obliteration of vascular lumen (*arrows*). Thrombus is also seen in many of the vessels

likely to involve vessel wall damage leading to endothelial activation and to chronic vascular remodelling. At the histological level, there is proliferation of the smooth muscle and endothelial cells in the small pulmonary arteries (Fig. 6.7).

Clinical Features

Shortness of breath on exertion is the most common presenting symptom, but this is not specific for pulmonary hypertension and may also be suggestive of chronic anemia or chronic lung disease. Angina, syncope, ascites and peripheral edema occur at later stages of the disease progression.

Mortality

Confirmed PHT is a risk factor for early mortality, but there are conflicting reports on risk of early death in patients with raised TRV. There was a significant increased mortality with TRV >2.5 m/s in the NIH cohort studied by Gladwin and co-workers in the United States, but this did not appear to be the case in the French cohort. In a UK cohort higher TRV values were associated with an increased risk of death but with a much lower mortality rate than reported in the NIH cohort. Furthermore, TRV was not an independent risk factor for death. Our own experience is that there is not a notable increase in deaths in patients with TRV between 2.5 and 2.9 m/s followed over the past decade.

Screening and Further Investigation

A screening protocol is desirable for early diagnosis of asymptomatic or mildly symptomatic patients. Cardiac catheterization is invasive and not suitable for screening, while echocardiography is non-invasive and relatively inexpensive.

An elevated TRV on echocardiography should normally be repeated to determine if it is consistently increased. However, echocardiography has a high false positive rate, and, in the French study, using a cut-off value of 2.5 m/s, a positive predictive value of only 25 %. This could be improved by using a value of 2.9 m/s, and combining with other tests such as a raised N-terminal pro Brain Natiuretic Peptide (NT pro-BNP) and/or the six minute walk test. There is a recent Practice Guideline published by the American Thoracic Society which we recommend for use in screening and diagnosis (Fig. 6.8). We question its recommendations for hydroxyurea in patients with TRV of 2.5 m/s. The premise on which this recommendation are made are currently not backed up by robust evidence. Screening should be done in the steady state as TRV will increase during an acute painful episode. For children, it is still unclear if raised TRV is associated with increased mortality and elevated TRV is often transient. Consequently, we do not recommend screening of asymptomatic patients <16 years.

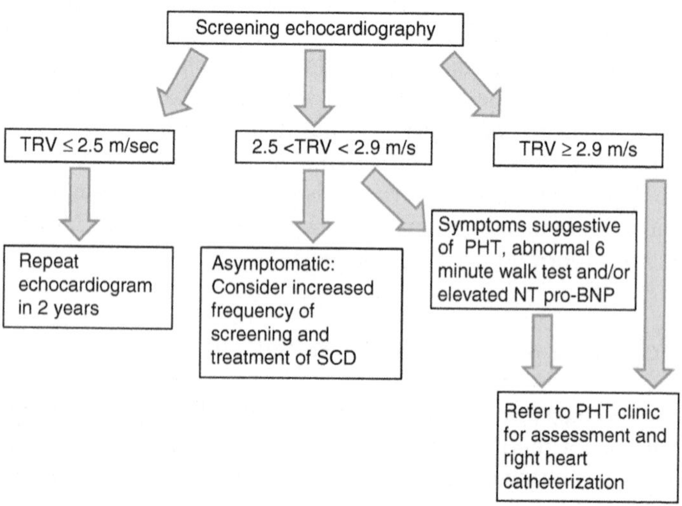

FIGURE 6.8 Algorithm for pulmonary hypertension screening

Management

Patients with clinical features of PHT require a specialist assessment. When the diagnosis is established, we recommend optimization of SCD control with hydroxyurea or transfusion therapy. The role of targeted pulmonary vascular therapies such as phosphodiesterase 5 inhibitors (e.g. sildenafil), prostacyclin analogues and endothelin-1-receptor antagonists (e.g. bosentan) is not clear. Both sildenafil and bosentan may be beneficial in some circumstances, but the limited clinical trials data currently available are not supportive. A randomized trial using sildenafil closed early because of an excess of adverse events (mostly pain) in the treatment group. A trial of bosentan failed to meet recruitment targets. There is anecdotal and indirect evidence that these therapies may be most beneficial in patients with precapillary PHT. Both agents should only be used with guidance from a pulmonary hypertension specialist. We believe that there is insufficient evidence to recommend treatment on the basis of a TR jet velocity of >2.5 m/s on its own, although there may be additional indications to support treatment in these individuals.

Asthma

Definition

Asthma has been defined in different ways. In some studies, it has relied on patient/parent report or physician diagnosis. In older children and adults the formal definition is based on demonstrated reversible airway obstruction on pulmonary function testing

Incidence

Asthma is seen in 17–22 % of children with SCD and is commoner than in age and race matched controls. Asthma prevalence does not seem to be increased in adults, but data is limited.

Pathophysiology

The association of childhood asthma with SCD is not understood at present. There is some evidence that airways obstruction is due to increased pulmonary capillary blood volume secondary to chronic anemia. Another suggestion is that it may be secondary to the chronic inflammatory state in the lungs induced by vaso-occlusion, reperfusion and free-radical generation.

Clinical Presentation

Children may present with typical symptoms of wheeze, chest pain and shortness of breath, which may be nocturnal or related to exercise. Alternatively symptoms of wheezing can be a feature of an acute painful episode or an infective episode. Asthma is a risk factor for acute chest syndrome, acute painful crises and for increased mortality in children.

Diagnosis

Diagnosis is based on symptoms and clinical findings. Children and parents should be questioned about symptoms of wheezing and chest examination should be performed in clinic and when presenting acutely unwell. Peak flow monitoring before and after the administration of bronchodilators is helpful in older children and adults. Respiratory function testing will show an obstructive abnormality and may show bronchial hyper-reactivity. Serum IgE levels, eosinophilia and allergen sensitivity are also helpful in supporting the diagnosis.

Management

Patients with a diagnosis of asthma should be managed jointly with a respiratory specialist. The management should include a regular review of asthma control and standard anti-asthma treatment should be used. Bronchodilators have an essential role in the management of acute chest syndrome in patients with a history of asthma or evidence of wheeze.

Chronic Sickle Lung Syndrome

Definition

Chronic sickle lung disease in SCD encompasses a variety of overlapping complications including pulmonary fibrosis and pulmonary hypertension. Chronic sickle lung syndrome has been used to describe a more specific clinical picture of a progressive, restrictive lung function deficit associated with fibrotic changes seen on high resolution CT scan of the chest. It is becoming increasingly clear that respiratory function abnormalities evolve over time in SCD. Young children are more likely to have an obstructive picture, but this is replaced by a progressive restrictive deficit in older children and adults. It is not yet clear how these pulmonary function abnormalities relate to the pathophysiology and long-term clinical complications of SCD, and chronic sickle lung syndrome is particularly poorly understood.

Incidence

Restrictive lung defects occur in over 70 % of adults in some studies, but are unusual in children less than ten years of age. A decrease in diffusion coefficient (DLCO) is also common in adults and is probably a sign of early interstitial lung disease. Daytime hypoxia (SaO_2 <94 %) is also common.

Clinical Features

Dyspnoea, fatigue, exercise limitation, hypoxia, dizziness and chest pain are suggestive symptoms in an adult, and the progressive nature may become apparent on regular outpatient review. These symptoms may be due to a variety of complications of SCD, and further assessment is needed to correlate with respiratory abnormalities. Chronic sickle lung syndrome may be associated with previous recurrent acute chest syndrome, but this is not always the case.

Diagnosis

A respiratory symptom review, oxygen saturation and physical examination of the chest should be part of regular out-patient assessment in adults, and part of the Annual Review. If there is evidence of progressive respiratory symptoms, or worsening hypoxia, further investigations should be arranged. These could include chest X ray, pulmonary function tests, echocardiography and sleep study. Arterial blood gases may be required to assess the need for home oxygen. High resolution CT scanning is the best method for demonstrating interstitial fibrotic lung disease, and the characteristic features in SCD include reticular abnormalities, and lobar volume loss (Fig. 6.9).

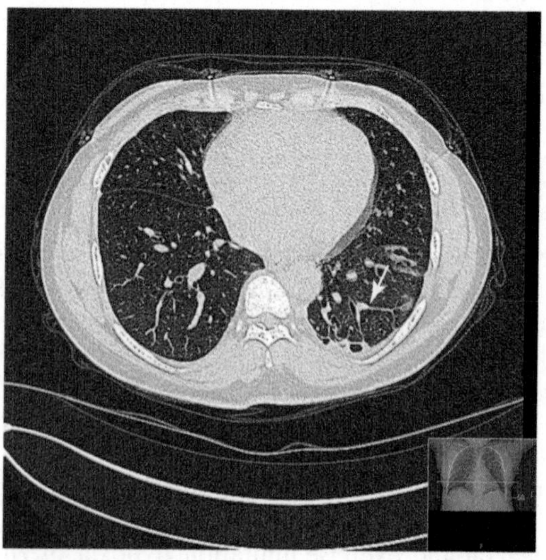

FIGURE 6.9 High resolution CT of chest showing fibrotic changes and traction bronchiectasis at L lung base (*arrow*), female age 40 with HbSS and history of chronic cough

Management

Joint management with a specialist in respiratory medicine is needed for severe cases. Patients may need counselling about smoking cessation and should ensure they are up to date with routine vaccinations including pneumococcal and annual influenza immunization. Home oxygen and bronchodilators may be indicated based on respiratory assessment. It is not clear to what extent chronic lung disease can be controlled by SCD-related therapies, however it is reasonable to consider hydroxyurea, particularly if there is a significant previous history of acute chest syndrome. Chronic transfusion may be considered, particularly if a low steady state hemoglobin is thought to be contributing to progressive hypoxemia.

Sleep Disordered Breathing and Hypoxemia

Definition

Sleep disordered breathing includes obstructive sleep apnea (OSA) and nocturnal hypoxemia. OSA is a documented obstruction in the upper airways during sleep. There are various technical definitions of OSA that relate to the different techniques of polysonography (Sleep Study) to measure air movement and respiratory effort. Hemoglobin oxygen saturation can also be measured overnight during a sleep study. Mean values of <94 % are generally considered abnormal in children with SCD. OSA and nocturnal hypoxemia can both occur simultantaneously.

Prevalence

Over 40 % of children and adolescents have nocturnal hypoxemia and 10–30 % have OSA. Nocturnal hypoxemia is seen in up to 60 % of adults with SCD. Both conditions are commonest in the HbSS genotype.

Pathophysiology

In young children OSA is often secondary to adenotonsillar hypertrophy. Overnight hypoxemia may be due to chronic lung disease or pulmonary hypertension, but may also related to artefactual low readings with altered wave length absorbance due to the abnormal haemoglobin molecule. In some cases, an extreme right shift in oxygen dissociation may contribute. These phenomena are not fully understood and often give rise to confusion in clinical assessment of hypoxemia.

Clinical Features

Patients with OSA may be asymptomatic or have symptoms of snoring and daytime somnolence. Obstructive sleep apnoea and overnight hypoxemia are associated with an increased risk of stroke, acute painful crises, pulmonary hypertension, renal dysfunction and priapism and have a negative impact on neuropsychological function and growth.

Investigation

Children presenting with symptoms of OSA require an urgent sleep study. Overnight oximetry cannot currently be recommended as a routine screening investigation in asymptomatic children outside the context of a clinical study. Children and adults with severe symptoms require examination of the upper airway and for those with severe hypoxemia and no obstruction, investigation for concurrent lung disease with CT of the chest, respiratory function testing and echocardiography should be considered.

Management

Children or adults with obstructive sleep apnoea confirmed on sleep study should be referred to an ENT surgeon for assessment of the upper airway and consideration of adenotonsillectomy. Nocturnal hypoxia unrelated to upper airway obstruction should be assessed by a respiratory physician, ideally in a multidisciplinary joint sickle cell/respiratory clinic. The efficacy, safety and acceptability of nocturnal CPAP and oxygen therapy are not yet established, but several trials are currently examining their potential roles.

Cardiac Abnormalities

In addition to PHT, SCD patients generally have elevated cardiac output and cardiomegaly. A significant proportion of patients investigated for PHT have a raised pulmonary capillary wedge pressure on cardiac catheterization, indicating left ventricular (LV) dysfunction. These abnormalities may be related to the long-term effect of chronic anemia, but there is also evidence from post-mortem studies of small vessel disease and local ischemic lesions in the myocardium, presumably related to vaso-occlusion. The prevalence and natural history of LV dysfunction in SCD is not well described at present, although it is likely to increase with an aging SCD population.

Investigations

Most adult patients are screened for PHT with echocardiography, and this will also identify significant left ventricular abnormalities. ECG may be unhelpful as nonspecific changes are often seen in SCD. Cardiac MRI is probably the optimal method for demonstrating localized wall dysfunction, ischemic lesions and myocardial perfusion defects.

Management

It is probably wise to transfuse patients who are severely anemic, hypoxemic and symptomatic with LV dysfunction. Although SCD patients do not seem to develop cardiac iron overload in the first few years of chronic transfusion, this may happen after prolonged transfusion and they will require iron chelation therapy to maintain iron balance. Less severely anemic patients could be managed with hydroxyurea. Control of hypertension and other risk factors for cardiac disease are also important.

Bibliography

Anim SO, Strunk RC, DeBaun M. Asthma morbidity and treatment in children with sickle cell disease. Expert Rev Respir Med. 2011;5(5):635–45.

Bellet PS, et al. Incentive spirometry to prevent acute pulmonary complications in sickle cell diseases. N Engl J Med. 1995;333:699–703.

Cabrita IZ, Mohammed A, Layton M, et al. The association between tricuspid regurgitation velocity and 5-year survival in a North West London population of patients with sickle cell disease in the United Kingdon. Br J Haem. 2013;162:400–8.

Gladwin MT, Sachdev V, Jison ML, et al. Pulmonary Hypertension as a Risk Factor for Death in Patients with Sickle Cell Disease. N Engl J Med. 2004;350(9):886–95.

Hargrave DR, Wade A, Evans JPM, Hewes DKM, Kirkham FJ. Nocturnal oxygen saturation and painful sickle cell crises in children. Blood. 2003;101(3):846–8.

Klings ES, Machado RF, Barst RJ, et al. An official American Thoracic Society clinical practice guideline: diagnosis, risk stratification and management of pulmonary hypertension of sickle cell disease. Am J Respir Crit Care Med. 2014;189(6):727–40.

Machado RF, Barst RJ, Yovetich NA, et al. Hospitalization for pain in patients with sickle cell disease treated with sildenafil for elevated TRV and low exercise capacity. Blood. 2011;118(4):855–64.

Parent F, Bachir D, Inamo J, Lionnet F, Driss F, Loko G, Habibi A, Bennani S, Savale L, Adnot S, Maitre B, Yaici A, Hajji L, O'Callaghan DS, Clerson P, Girot R, Galacteros F, Simonneau G.

A Hemodynamic Study of Pulmonary Hypertension in Sickle Cell Disease. N Engl J Med. 2011;365:44–53.

Vichinsky EP, et al. Acute chest syndrome in sickle cell disease: clinical presentation and cause. Blood. 1997;89:1787–92.

Vichinsky EP, et al. Causes and outcomes of the acute chest syndrome in sickle cell disease. N Engl J Med. 2000;342:1855–65.

Vij R, Machado RF. Pulmonary Complications of Hemoglobinopathies. Chest. 2010;138(4):973–83.

Voskaridou E, Chirstoulas D, Terpos E. Sickle cell disease and the heart: review of the current literature. Br J Haematol. 2012;157:664–73.

Chapter 7
Neurological Complications

Introduction

The brain is particularly vulnerable to ischemia and an important aim of management is the prevention of cognitive as well as physical disability due to progressive brain damage. Patients who are at risk of neurological complications are not necessarily those who experience frequent painful crises.

The important acute and chronic neurological complications of SCD are presented in Table 4.1 and the anatomy of the major intra-cerebral arteries indicating common sites of vascular damage in Figs. 7.1 and 7.2.

Ischemic Lesions

Definitions

For clinical diagnosis, we recommend using definitions developed for use in clinical trials. These criteria require confirmation by a specialist neurologist and neuroradiologist.

J. Howard, P. Telfer, *Sickle Cell Disease in Clinical Practice*, In Clinical Practice, DOI 10.1007/978-1-4471-2473-3_7,

Acute Ischemic Stroke (AIS)

History of acute neurological deficit consistent with an arterial territory lesion, and with an acute ischemic lesion in the corresponding vascular territory on magnetic resonance imaging (MRI). Very occasionally, an ischemic lesion is not visible on MRI. This would still be diagnosed as AIS if the neurological deficit was persisting.

Transient Ischemic Attack (TIA)

History of acute neurological deficit lasting less than 24 hours consistent with a lesion in an arterial territory, without a residual neurological deficit, and with no evidence of an acute ischemic lesion on MRI.

Silent Cerebral Infarction (SCI)

Ischemic lesion on MRI (at least 3mm in diameter, seen in two planes) with no clinically detectable neurological deficit.

Etiology and Pathophysiology

Cerebral Ischemia

This is a consequence of failure to maintain adequate brain perfusion. It is assumed that compensatory blood flow around the Circle of Willis is inadequate in the presence of acute anemia, chronic vessel wall damage, and acute vaso-occlusion due to sickled red cells and/or thrombus formation. Ischemic damage is most common in the distribution of the middle cerebral artery (MCA), the watershed region of restricted perfusion between the MCA and the anterior cerebral artery (ACA) or between the MCA and posterior cerebral artery (PCA) (Figs. 7.1 and 7.2).

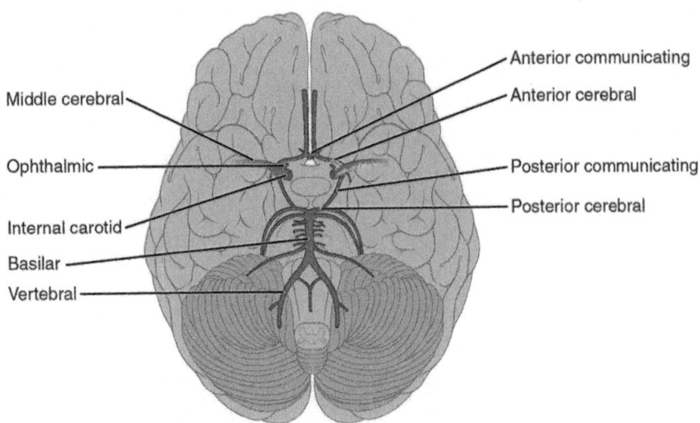

FIGURE 7.1 The arterial supply of the brain. The common sites of stenotic or occlusive lesions seen in children with SCD are shown (*yellow hatched*)

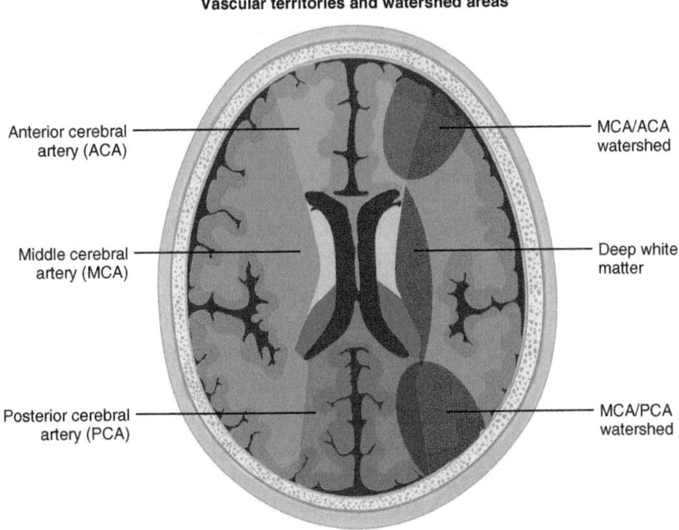

FIGURE 7.2 Transverse section through the cerebral hemispheres at the level of lateral ventricles showing the vascular territories of major cerebral arteries (*left side*) and 'watershed' areas at the borders of these vascular territories which are susceptible to ischemic damage (*right side*)

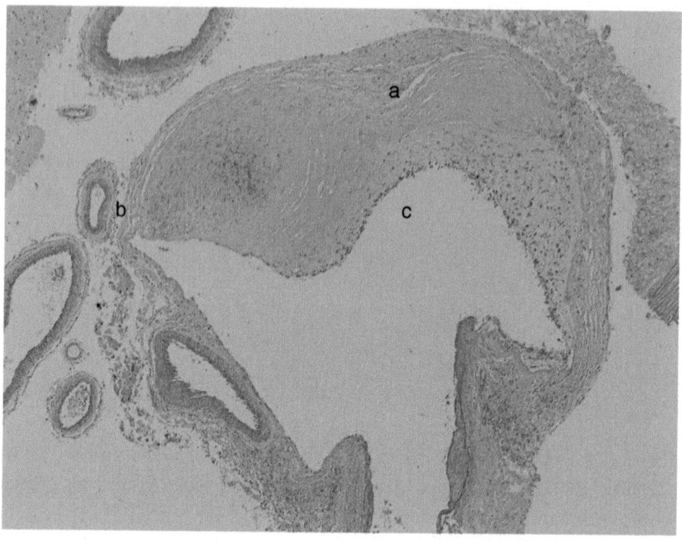

FIGURE 7.3 Post mortem histological section through parts of a major intracerebral artery showing areas of thickening (*a*) and thinning (*b*) of the vessel wall. The vessel lumen is also narrowed (*c*)

Cerebral Artery Vasculopathy

Acute ischemic stroke is often (but not always) associated with an arterial vasculopathy characterized by stenotic or occlusive lesions in the large vessels, most commonly the internal carotid artery (ICA) proximal MCA and ACA (Figs. 7.1 and 7.2). The posterior cerebral artery (PCA) and basilar arteries are less commonly and less severely affected. Histological examination of the vessel wall shows intramural thrombus which is often organized and re-canalized. The vessel wall is damaged with endothelial disruption, duplication of the internal elastic lamina and scarring of the tunica media (Fig. 7.3). These vascular lesions often arise at areas of turbulence. It is here that shearing forces caused by abnormal sickled red cells flowing over the endothelium are

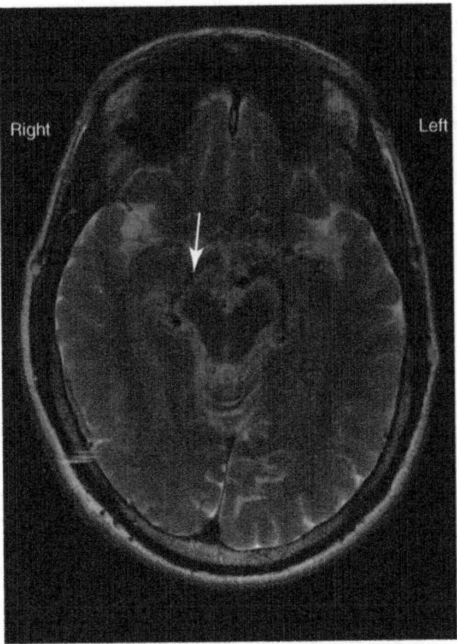

FIGURE 7.4 T2 weighted cerebral MRI of adult male. The MCA is occluded and not visible on the *right side*. Moyamoya vessels in section are seen as numerous black dots (flow voids) in the region of the midbrain (*arrow*)

most likely to cause physical damage and provoke inflammation.

Vasculopathy can be progressive, leading to large vessel occlusion and new vessel formation. Moyamoya is a term used to describe a particular appearance of abnormal vasculature with vessel dilatation and new vessel formation. Moyamoya vessel formation implies a worse prognosis for stroke, silent ischemia and cerebral hemorrhage. Moyamoya changes are visible on cerebral MRI (Fig. 7.4) and Magnetic Resonance Angiography (MRA) although direct angiography is required for confirmation of findings and for planning surgical or invasive radiological intervention (Fig. 7.5a, b).

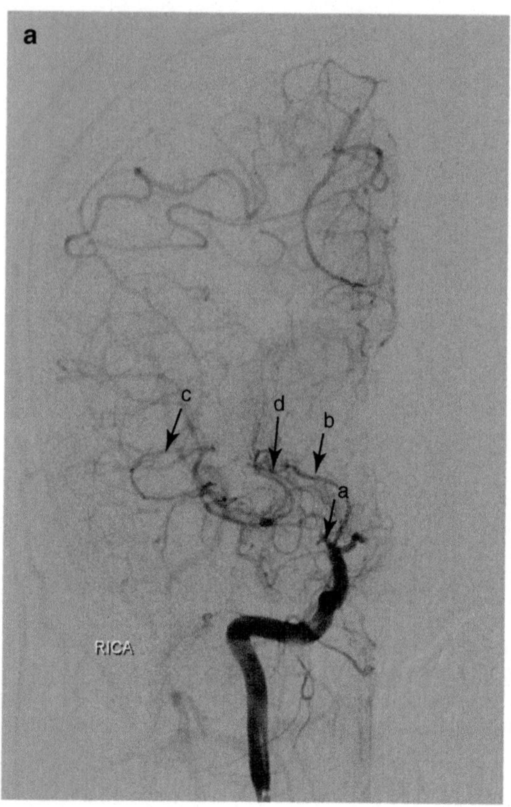

FIGURE 7.5 (**a**) Moyamoya in a 20 year old woman with HbSS. Digital subtraction angiogram with contrast injection into the right internal carotid artery. The right middle cerebral artery is occluded near its origin (*a*), distal to the proximal lenticulostriate artery (*b*), which is filling the distal middle cerebral artery and its tributaries (*c*) through the distal lenticulostriate arteries (*d*). (**b**) Digital subtraction angiogram with contrast injection into the left internal carotid artery (same patient as a). In contrast to the right side, this shows normal MCA (*a*) but near-absent filling of the left anterior cerebral artery. Very faint filling of the ACA is seen (*b*) through moyamoya collaterals (*c*). *RICA* right internal carotid artery, *LICA* left internal carotid artery

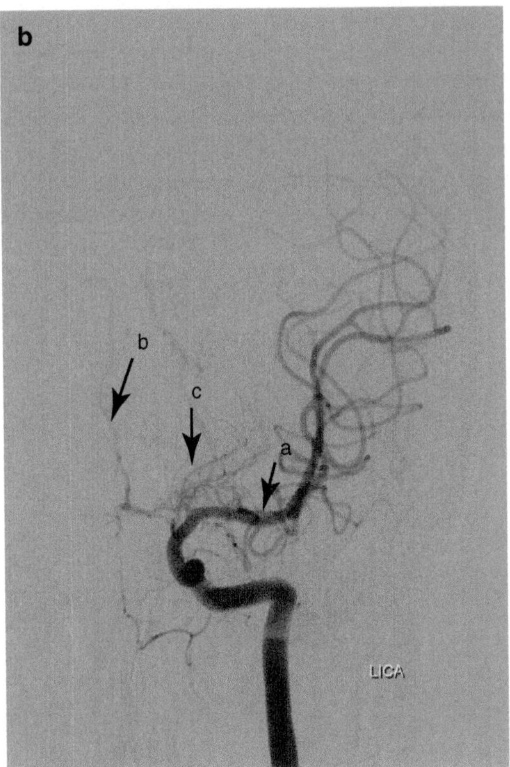

FIGURE 7.5 (continued)

Vasculopathy can also affect the carotid and vertebral arteries in the neck (Fig. 7.6). Lesions in the cervical portion of the ICA have been associated with ischemic stroke involving the territories of the MCA and ACA, as well as progressive silent ischemia in the anterior watershed distribution.

Radiological Investigation and Findings

Cerebral magnetic resonance imaging (MRI) is the investigation of choice for suspected ischemic lesions. These appear as hyper-intense (white) areas on T2-weighted sequences. FLAIR (Fluid Attenuated Inverse Relaxation) increases the conspicuity of ischemic lesions as the fluid signal from CSF in the ventricles and around the brain is nulled out and appears hypo-dense (black). T2 FLAIR images are often used for accurate determination of the position and size of infarcts (Fig. 7.7a) and are essential for diagnosis of silent ischaemia.

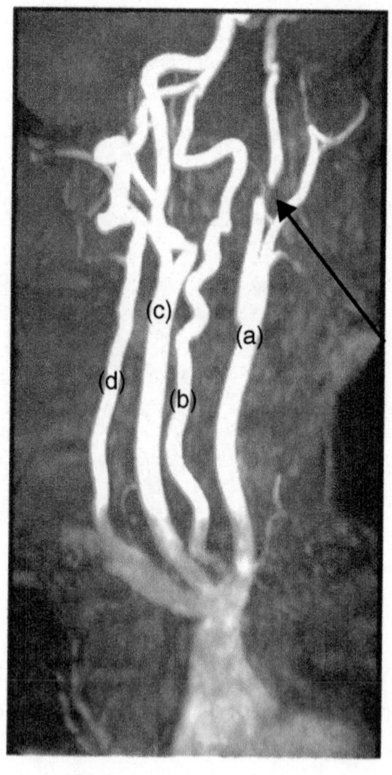

FIGURE 7.6 MRA of major cervical arteries. Oblique view showing occlusion of left ICA just beyond the bifurcation of the common carotid artery (*arrow*). The left common carotid (*a*), left vertebral artery (*b*), right common carotid (*c*), and right vertebral arteries (*d*) can be seen. A common incidental finding is abnormal tortuosity of the vertebral arteries

In the acute setting, diffusion weighted imaging is useful for identifying areas of acute cell swelling in the early stages of ischemia (Fig. 7.7b).

Computerized tomography (CT) is commonly used in emergency departments and is the preferred imaging method

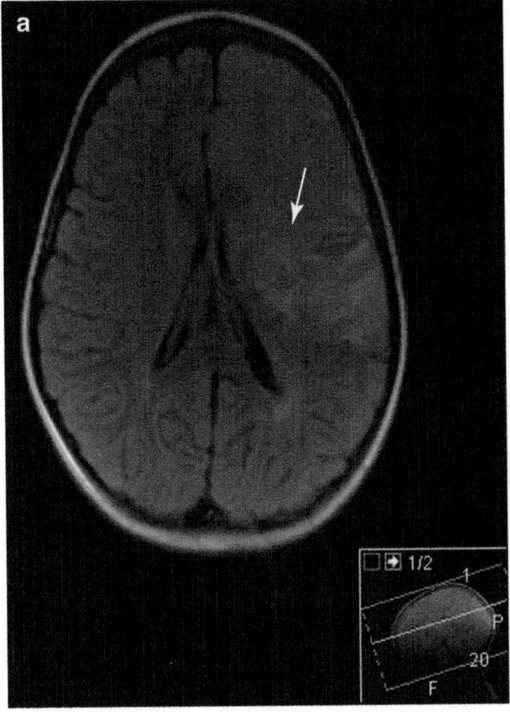

FIGURE 7.7 Cerebral MRI of a 4 year old child presenting with R hemiparesis resulting from an acute ischaemic stroke with left ICA occlusion. (**a**) T2 FLAIR image showing a large high intensity lesion in the territory of the ACA and MCA with involvement of the cortex and basal ganglia (*arrow*). (**b**) Diffusion weighted image (DWI) showing high signal in the same areas, consistent with acute ischemia (*arrow*)

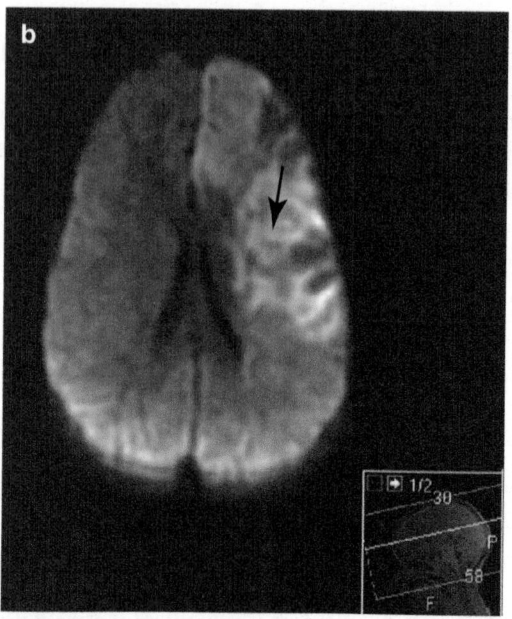

FIGURE 7.7 (continued)

for acute cerebral haemorrhage. For suspected acute ischemic events, head CT should be followed by magnetic resonance imaging.

Magnetic resonance angiography (MRA) is an important non-invasive method for demonstrating stenotic or occlusive lesions in the large arterial vessels of the head and neck. MRA identifies reduced or turbulent blood flow within the vessel lumen and is therefore an indirect method of demonstrating stenosis or occlusion. More refined MRI techniques can be used to image the vessel wall directly (for instance to demonstrate a dissection or intra-luminal thrombus).

CT Angiography and Direct Four Vessel Contrast Angiography

These techniques are preferred for accurate determination of the location and size of vascular lesions and aneurysms. They are important for defining the vascular anatomy and extent of collateral flow prior to undertaking surgical bypass procedures or interventional neuroradiology.

Acute Ischemic Stroke (AIS)

Clinical Presentation

Patients may present with typical features of stroke: hemiparesis or single limb weakness, hemi-facial droop, hemi-anopia or dysphasia. Sometimes the presentation is less obvious, with transient diminished motor function, loss of consciousness, confusion, or behavioural change. Usually the presentation is purely neurological, but AIS can also be a complication of a severe vaso-occlusive crisis, most commonly a severe acute chest syndrome, or an acute anemic event. In the presence of an antecedent crisis, the risk of recurrent stroke is lower. There have also been reports of events occurring after varicella zoster, parvovirus, and other acute infections.

Assessment and Investigations

Apart from a detailed neurological examination, repeated periodically to determine progression or regression of neurological signs, it is important to assess for evidence of additional sickle complications, as well as for infection, obstructive sleep apnea, abnormalities in blood pressure, and oxygen saturation. Laboratory tests (Table 4.3) are important for

TABLE 7.1 Recommended investigation of acute neurological event

Investigation	Purpose
CT brain	Emergency diagnosis of AHS if MRI unavailable at presentation. (Ischaemic changes may not be apparent in the first few hours after the event)
Cerebral MRI: T1- and T2-weighted, FLAIR and DWI.	Confirmation and anatomical localization of acute hemorrhagic and ischemic stroke. Exclusion of other acute neurological disorders including PRES
Cerebral and cervical MRA. Fat-saturated imaging of cervical ICA. Magnetic resonance venogram.	Demonstration of intracerebral arterial occlusion(s). Demonstration of chronic vasculopathic lesions (e.g. moyamoya). Further investigation of suspected extracranial arterial stenosis/occlusion/ dissection or cerebral venous sinus thrombosis if clinically indicated
Echocardiography	Exclusion of intra-cardiac thrombus and patent foramen ovale

excluding an acute anemic event, for compatibility testing and for determining HbS% prior to urgent exchange transfusion. Low steady state hemoglobin, and raised white cell count are risk factors for AIS, but do not guide treatment in the acute situation. Radiological investigations recommended for investigating an acute neurological event are listed in Table 7.1.

Incidence

The incidence is highest in HbSS, and much lower in HbSC and HbS β thalassaemia. For acute infarctive stroke, the highest incidence rate is in children in the age range 2 to 9 years (between 0.5 and 1 per 100 patient years follow-up). The rate is also high in adults over the age of 40. Implementation of TCD screening programmes has significantly reduced the incidence of AIS as we shall see later in this chapter.

Management

AIS is a medical emergency. The objectives of treatment are to minimise ischemic damage, improve perfusion of viable tissue and prevent recurrence. Initial management should ensure hemodynamic stabilization, adequate hydration, and normalization of oxygenation saturation. Although there are no trials evaluating transfusion in AIS, exchange transfusion has become standard practice with the objective of optimizing Hb level and reducing HbS percentage urgently. If the Hb is <70 g/l top-up transfusion should precede exchange. The target HbS is <30 %, and Hb level should not be allowed to exceed 110 g/l.

There have been no trials evaluating the use of aspirin, anticoagulation or thrombolysis in acute management of AIS. These interventions are not necessarily beneficial, since the pathophysiology of AIS in SCD is different from thromboembolic stroke in the elderly, where these treatments are well established. We recommend that adults are considered on an individual basis if presenting within the therapeutic window for thrombolysis.

In the UK, adult SCD patients could be managed on a specialized acute stroke unit, and it is advisable to formulate a local protocol with stroke physicians for imaging investigations, acute treatment and rehabilitation. AIS in older patients may be related to cerbrovascular risk factors which apply to the general population. These patients should be discussed with a stroke physician to decide if sickle or non-sickle risk factors are predominant and whether they should be treated initially with thrombolysis or exchange transfusion.

During recovery from the acute effects of a stroke, longer-term rehabilitation needs to be discussed and planned. The most severe cases are physically disabled and wheel-chair bound. They are also likely to have severe cognitive deficits, which will have a profound effect on their education, social life and employment prospects. Furthermore, the support network within the family may not be strong. This is a situation where effective engagement of multi-disciplinary support is very important. A range of specialist interventions can be helpful, including physiotherapy, psychology, speech and

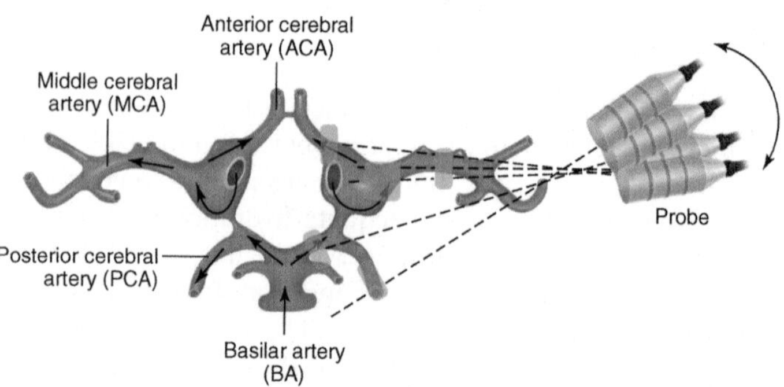

FIGURE 7.8 Transcranial Doppler probe positioning and angulation to detect flow signals. Flow velocities from the proximal portions of the Middle cerebral artery (MCA) and anterior cerebral artery (ACA) are measured with small changes in angulation of the probe positioned over the temporal part of the skull. Flow velocities from the posterior cerebral arteries (PCA) and basilar artery (BA) can also be obtained

language therapy, occupational therapy, social work and support services for special educational needs. These interventions can be planned and co-ordinated through a multi-disciplinary case conference in which parents and carers are involved.

Primary Prevention: Transcranial Doppler (TCD) Ultrasonography

TCD ultrasonography can be used to measure blood velocity in the large intra-cerebral arteries. It is suitable for detecting early vascular lesions because blood flows at increased velocity through a stenosed vessel. The segments most prone to stenosis in SCD (terminal ICA, and first segments of MCA and ACA) can be insonated in the axis of flow by adjusting the angle of the ultrasound probe at the trans-temporal window (Fig. 7.8). Distal to a significant stenosis, velocity is usually attenuated. TCD screening was initially validated using a non-imaging scanning method, which requires careful positioning and angulation of the probe to identify the maximal audible

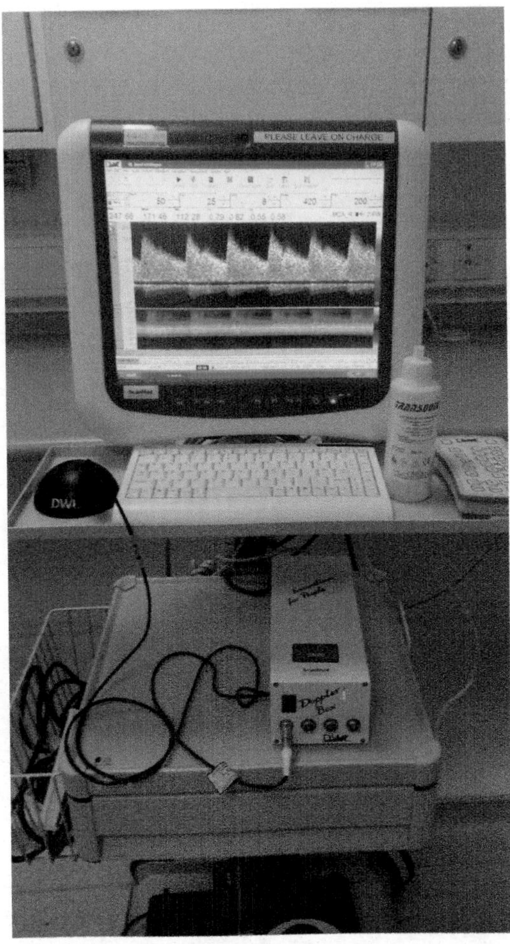

FIGURE 7.9 One of the non-imaging transcranial Doppler ultrasound scanners used in our service

doppler frequency. In TCD screening programs, scanning is either done using non-imaging equipment (Fig. 7.9) or duplex colour Doppler mapping systems (imaging TCD). Although earlier comparative studies suggested that imaging TCD was under-estimating maximal velocities, this now appears to be corrected by optimal allignment of the the imaging probe.

Time averaged mean of maximal velocity (TAMMV) of 200 cm/sec or more is often (but not always) associated with a stenotic vascular lesion demonstrable on MRA (Fig. 7.10). In the Medical College of Georgia (MCG) Cohort Study, children

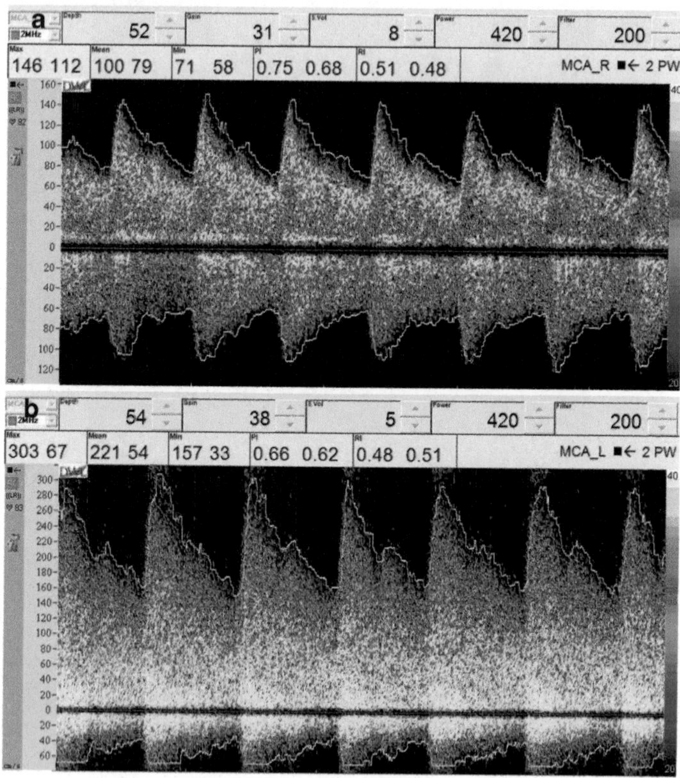

FIGURE 7.10 (**a**) Normal TCD spectrogram at a depth of 52 mm in a 10-year-old child. There are simultaneous signals from MCA (upward signal, towards the probe) and ACA (downward signal, away from the probe). The time averaged mean velocity in the MCA is 100 cm/s (normal). (**b**) Abnormal Doppler spectrogram in a 10-year-old child with cerebral vasculopathy showing time averaged mean velocity of 221 cm/s in the proximal MCA at a depth of 54 mm (**c**). MRA showing Circle of Willis in the same patient as (**b**). There are flow voids in the proximal MCA (*arrow a*) and ACA (*arrow b*) indicating severe stenotic lesions

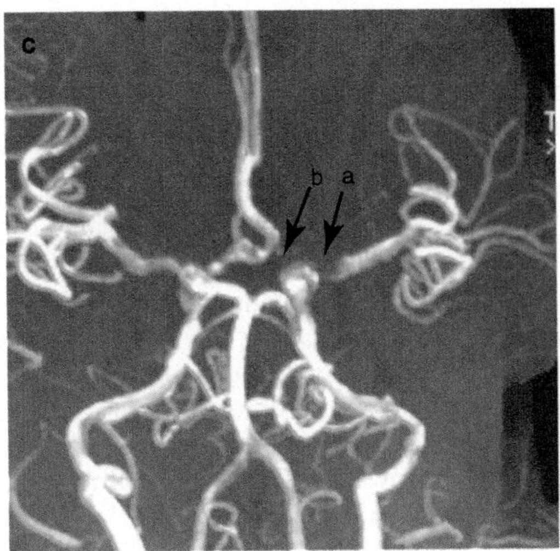

FIGURE 7.10 (continued)

with TAMMV confirmed at over 200 cm/sec had a high risk of stroke (40 % over 3 years follow-up) and these velocities were classified as abnormal. Those with TAMMV of 170 to 199 cm/sec had a lower risk of stroke (7 %) and were classified as 'Conditional'. Those with a TAMMV of less than 170 had the lowest risk (2 %) and were classified as 'Standard risk'. This system for categorizing scans has become widely accepted and used in the clinical setting.

In the STOP trial, children with confirmed abnormal TCD were randomized to transfusion or standard care. The trial was terminated early because of the significant treatment effect. Children randomised to transfusions had a 91 % reduction in stroke risk. Over the past ten years it has become routine to offer TCD scanning to children with HbSS and other severe genotypes (excluding HbSC and HbS β^+ thalassemia) every year from 2 to 16 years of age. Children with confirmed abnormal TCD are offered regular transfusion (top-up or exchange) for an indefinite period to maintain HbS <30 %.

In practice, this often leads to a difficult discussion, as many of the children with abnormal TCD are not severely affected by acute vaso-occlusive crises and parents may be reluctant to consider such a major treatment intervention when their child seems to be well.

Concurrent with implementation of TCD screening, the incidence of stroke has diminished significantly. In California, there was an abrupt fall in the years 1998–2000. Reports from single centers with well established programmes indicate an approximate tenfold reduction in AIS incidence to about 0.1 per 100 patient years follow-up.

In the UK, recommendations for TCD screening were published in 2009 and summarized in a flowchart (Fig. 7.11). There is a degree of operator dependence in TCD screening and the possibility of both false positive and negative results in inexperienced hands. Consequently, quality assurance of TCD scanning is required. Currently, in the absence of a national quality assurance scheme in the UK, a local quality assurance policy should be developed, including training and assessment of the continuing competency of practitioners.

Important questions still to be answered about management of children with abnormal TCD include

- Is it possible to refine the assessment of stroke risk in children with abnormal TCD?
- What is the minimum duration of transfusion required for protection? STOP2 attempted to answer this with randomization to discontinuation of regular transfusions in selected patients after 2 years. The trial was stopped early because of a significant rate of relapse to abnormal TCD or stroke in the non-transfused arm. The current recommendation is that transfusions cannot be safely discontinued during childhood.
- Is hydroxyurea an effective alternative to long-term transfusion? This question will be answered by the TWiTCH trial, a randomised controlled trial of continuing transfusion versus hydroxyurea in children who have normalised TCD velocities after at least one year of transfusions. The study end point is a composite of (i) reversion to abnormal TCD velocity and (ii) stroke.

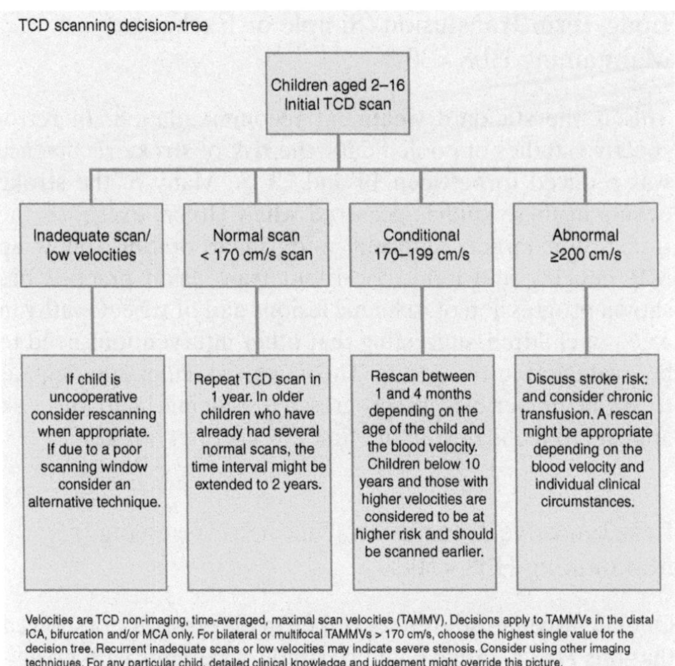

FIGURE 7.11 NHS TCD scanning protocol (from Antenatal and Neonatal Screening Programmes: Transcranial Doppler Scanning for Children with Sickle Cell Disease, Standards and Guidance, 2009)

Secondary Prevention

The risk of recurrent AIS has been reported between 47 and 93 %. Whilst there may be relatively little overt residual deficit after a first episode, progressive motor deficits and severe intellectual decline are inevitable with recurrent ischemic events. To avoid progressive neuro-disability, all patients should be considered for long-term preventive treatment after first AIS. Currently, there are several treatment options which could be considered:

Long-Term Transfusion (Simple or Exchange) Maintaining HbS <30 %

This is the standard treatment recommendation. In retrospective studies of pooled data, the risk of stroke recurrence was reduced to between 14 and 23 %. Many of the stroke events in these studies occurred when HbS% exceeded the transfusion target. A recent study incorporating follow-up MR imaging and more consistent transfusion practice has shown progression of ischemic lesions and of vasculopathy in 45 % of children, suggesting that other interventions need to be evaluated in this group. Those with vasculopathy appear to be at higher risk of progressive ischemia, and the risk appears to be highest in the first 2 years after stroke.

Less Intensive Transfusion (Simple or Exchange) Maintaining HbS <50 %

One single center study undertaken in the pre-MR era showed that this HbS% target could be used for patients with no evidence of recurrent stroke or TIA after 4 or 5 years of intensive transfusion. Annual transfusion volume and iron loading were significantly reduced after an average 7 years follow-up. There have been no controlled trials comparing different HbS% targets and it is not established whether patients on this regime are protected against progressive vasculopathy and silent ischemic lesions. We would not recommend this protocol for those with severe vasculopathy on MR or a history of TIAs. Annual follow-up MR scans should be done to exclude progressive ischemia or vasculopathy.

Hydroxyurea

It is often difficult to sustain a long-term transfusion programme. Situations where alternatives may need to be considered include: difficult venous access, erratic attendances for scheduled transfusion, red cell allo-immunization and uncontrolled transfusional iron overload. Ware and colleagues proposed that hydroxyurea could significant protect against recurrent stroke, while enhancing hemoglobin levels sufficiently to enable regular venesection. The benefits from venesection include reduction in hematocrit, which might improve microvascular blood flow, and reduction of transfusional iron overload. Using a protocol which included initial overlapping of transfusions and hydroxyurea and an escalation to achieve maximal tolerated dose, the stroke rate in a pilot study was 3.7 per 100 patient years (within the range of reported recurrence rate in patients on regular transfusion). Unexpectedly, these benefits were not realized in an RCT (the SWiTCH trial) designed to test non-inferiority of hydroxyurea plus venesections versus transfusion plus iron chelation. There was a significant excess of strokes in the hydroxyurea plus venesection arm (10 % vs 0 %) and no apparent benefit in reduction of iron overload. The trial authors concluded that transfusion and chelation remain a better way of managing children with SCD, stroke, and iron overload. Despite the negative results, we think there is sufficient evidence from the published literature to consider hydroxyurea with or without venesection in cases where transfusion therapy is not suitable (e.g. severe alloimmunization, recurrent transfusion reactions) and possibly in patients who have remained free from progressive ischemia and vasculopathy after at least 5 years of regular transfusion and are judged to be at relatively low risk of recurrence.

Vasculosurgical Interventions to Improve Cerebral Perfusion

Surgical revascularization has been recommended for patients who have recurrent AIS, TIA and/or progressive vasculopathy who are not stabilized during chronic transfusion therapy. There has been limited experience with this approach, and no controlled trials. The most common procedure is Encephaloduroarteriosynangiosis (EDAS) which aims to encourage revascularization and improve cerebral blood flow by transposing an arterial flap from the scalp onto the surface of the brain. Reports from case series suggest some benefit in improving perfusion and reducing recurrence, but some patients had new ischemic lesions on follow-up. We recommend that these patients should be discussed and assessed in a specialized neurovascular surgical unit. Four vessel angiography would be required in all cases in order to delineate the vascular anatomy and plan intervention.

Allogeneic Bone Marrow Transplantation (BMT)

If a histocompatible sibling donor is available, BMT is probably the treatment of choice for children with AIS. The benefits include cure of SCD and avoidance of an indefinite chronic transfusion programme with all its problems. The risks of BMT are discussed in Chap. 18. Early experience indicated an increased risk of acute neurological events during the peri-transplant period. This risk has been significantly reduced by careful attention to levels of Hb, HbS%, platelet count, blood pressure, and by using prophylactic anti-epileptics. Patients followed in the longer term have remained stroke-free and there appears to be stabilization and possibly an improvement in vasculopathy. More data is needed on long-term follow-up post-BMT, including documentation of serial MR imaging in patients with prior ischemic lesions and vasculopathy, to confirm these findings.

Silent Cerebral Infarction (SCI)

MR studies of stroke-free children with HbSS have shown ischemic lesions which are not apparent on neurological examination, often less extensive than in those with AIS and often with no evidence of vasculopathy. These silent ischemic lesions tend to be single, multiple, or occasionally confluent areas of infarction in the deep white matter, most commonly in the anterior watershed region (Fig. 7.12). SCI is associated with frontal and pre-frontal dysfunction and reduced IQ. The cognitive problems affect concentration, short term memory and processing of complex information. These deficits become apparent in the later stages of primary education when demands on the intellect are increasing.

The prevalence of SI lesions increases during childhood from about 10 % in infants to 28 % by the age of 5 and 37 % by the age of 15.

There is a significant risk of progressive cerebral ischemia in children with SCI, including new and enlarging SCI lesions, and acute stroke. The SIT (Silent Infarct Transfusion) Trial

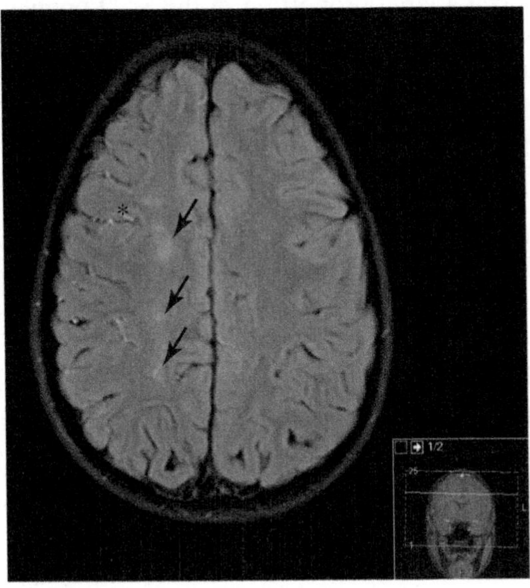

FIGURE 7.12 Cerebral MRI (T2 FLAIR) of 8 years old boy with HbSS showing characteristic appearance of silent ischemia in the deep white matter of the right cerebral hemisphere (arrows). Abnormal vessels are seen on the surface of the cortex (*) indicating pial neovascularization. This child had a severe stenosis in the right internal carotid artery

was an international, multicentre randomised controlled trial in which children with HbSS aged 5 to 15 years were screened with cerebral MRI. Those with SCI lesions were offered randomization to transfusion or observation. Comparing children with and without SCI at screening, the risk factors for SCI were low steady state Hb and higher systolic blood pressure. The trial results showed a significant reduction in the composite end point of progressive SCI and overt acute stroke for children on transfusion. In the intention to treat analysis, most of the difference between the groups was due to a reduction in stroke rather than SCI. At the time of writing, the implications of these results are still being evaluated. There are many questions about how to implement the findings into clinical practice. It will be challenging to offer MR screening to all HbSS children and to offer long-term transfusion to such a large proportion of the SCD population. The authors of the final SIT report recommended a screening MR scan in pre-school children, in order to identify children affected at an early age who can be targeted for educational and medical intervention. These children would usually require sedation for an MR scan, and this entails some risks as well as further resources for service provision.

Children identified with SCI whose performance at school is below expectation should be referred for neuropsychometric assessment, and results discussed with teachers and special education needs co-ordinators. Specific advice can be given to optimise learning. such as:

- Sitting near the front of the class to avoid distraction
- Giving more time to undertake learning activities
- Learning to break down complex information into simpler units

MR studies in adults have also shown the typical SCI lesions seen in children but the prevalence has been variable. Other findings include encephalomalacia, lacuna infarcts, and cortical atrophy. It is not yet clear how these lesions relate to the long-term natural history of SCI, and clarification will require long-term MR surveillance studies. Adults may also have evidence of cognitive impairment affecting the same domains of functioning seen in children with SCI. Neuropsychometric assessment can be helpful in demonstrating memory and processing deficits and might be used to assist requesting support for college studies, examinations and work planning.

Acute Hemorrhagic Stroke (AHS)

AHS includes intracerebral, intraventricular, subdural and subarachnoid hemorrhage (SAH).

Incidence

Incidence rates of AHS are high in adolescents and young adults with HbSS (approximately 0.4 per 100 patient years follow-up). It is interesting that this age range is relatively spared from AIS - the explanation for which is not clear. About 9 % of adults with HbSS have an aneurysm on routine MRA screening, which is at least twice the rate in the general population. It is possible that TCD screening and primary AIS prevention will inhibit the development and progression of vasculopathic lesions and hence reduce the risk of AHS in the future, but there is no evidence for this at present.

Etiology

Vasculopathy underlies many cases, and AHS may be a complication in patients with moyamoya vessel formation. Relative hypertension is another risk factor. Patients who present with SAH are often found to have single or multiple aneurysms in the anterior or vertebro-basilar circulations. AHS can also be a complication of venous sinus thrombosis. Subdural hemorrhage may occur apparently spontaneously although the possibility of non-accidental injury must be investigated in young children.

Clinical Presentation

Clinical features have been described in historical case series, notably a retrospective comparison of cases of AIS and AHS from two pediatric institutions in the USA. Children and young adults with AHS present most commonly with headache and reduced level of consciousness. This is typically preceded by an inter-current severe complication (e.g. hepatic or renal impairment), sometimes leading to over-transfusion (high Hb) and coagulopathy. Presentation with hemiparesis and focal neurological signs is less common. Seizures were observed in both AIS and AHS. AHS is also one of the causes of a sudden death outside of hospital.

Diagnostic Criteria

Diagnosis of AHS requires radiological demonstration of intracranial blood. In the case of SAH, clinical history of sudden onset severe headache and signs of meningism associated with xanthrochromia in cerebrospinal fluid is sufficient for diagnosis.

Investigations

CT is suitable for diagnosis of acute intra-cerebral hemorrhage and is usually the first available imaging modality in the emergency department. Lumbar puncture should be done for suspected SAH if the initial CT is negative. If intracranial haemorrhage is present, CT angiography of the intracranial vessels should be performed to identify aneurysms or moya moya vasculopathy.

Treatment

In most cases patients should be managed on a specialized neurosurgical or high dependency unit with medical input from the SCD specialist team. Neurological complications such as seizures or coma should be managed according to standard protocols. Intensive monitoring is required with careful control of blood pressure, normalization of oxygenation and hydration. Optimization of hemoglobin level to about 80 g/l is recommended, but it is important not to over-transfuse. Exchange transfusion is usually performed, especially if neurosurgery or interventional radiology is being considered, and this should be done carefully, maintaining isovolemia throughout the procedure.

Aneurysms may be treated either by surgical ablation, or coil embolization depending on size and position. In our experience, coiling of aneurysms has been very successful (Figs. 7.13 and 7.14).

Screening and Prevention

Currently, there is no reliable screening method to identify patients at high risk of AHS, but some centers are screening young adults with cerebral MRI and MRA in order to detect those with aneurysm or moyamoya. Patients with single or multiple arterial aneurysms, or moyamoya vessels identified on MR or direct angiography are at increased risk of AHS. In these cases, interventional radiology or surgical revascularization may be considered to reduce the risk of a future event.

Venous Sinus Thrombosis (VST)

This is an under-recognised condition which may occur at any age, including neonates, and is associated with significant mortality as well as morbidity if untreated. Risk factors include infection, dehydration, trauma and anemia.

Clinical Features

Patients with acute illness, including meningitis and other infections, are at risk particularly if fluid intake has been inadequate. Headache, behavioural abnormalities and seizure may precede deterioration in conscious level and there may be focal neurological signs.

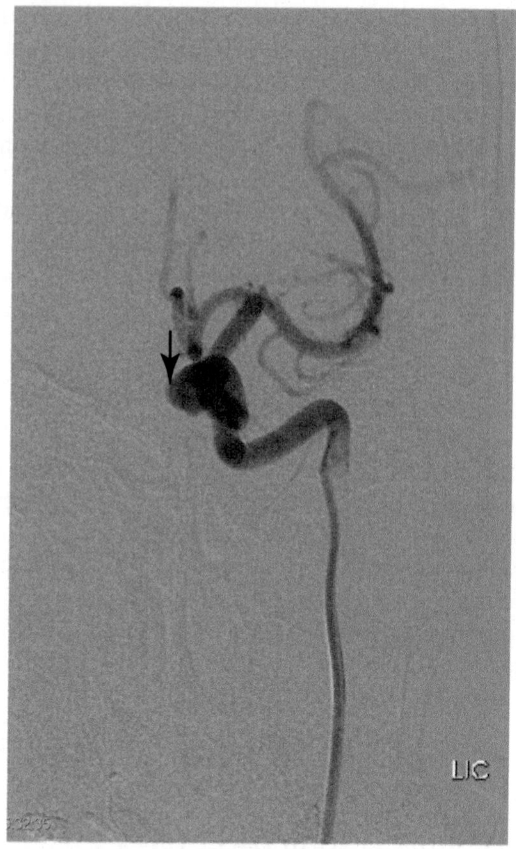

FIGURE 7.13 Digital subtraction angiogram with contrast injection into the left internal carotid artery in a 25-year-old man with HbSS showing an aneurysm just distal to the cavernous segment of the internal carotid artery (*arrow*)

Pathophysiology

Thrombosis may occur in the superficial (superior sagittal sinus, transverse sinus) or the deep (straight sinus, vein of Galen) cerebral venous system and may propagate if the precipitants (e.g. infection and dehydration) are not reversed and the thrombosis remains untreated. Spontaneous recana-

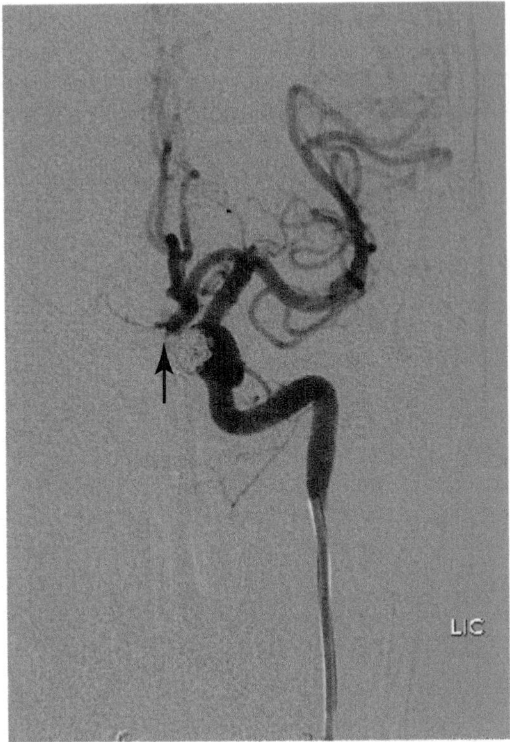

FIGURE 7.14 Following coil embolization of the aneurysm (*arrow*). The vasculature beyond the lesion (distal ICA, MCA and ACA) is patent

lisation may occur relatively quickly, making diagnosis difficult unless venography is undertaken early. Risk factors for recurrence include age over 2 years, non-recanalisation of the venous system and non-treatment during at risk situations.

Investigations

On CT or MRI, venous infarction typically involves the parietal, occipital and frontal lobes and the thalami: there may be extensive brain swelling. Venous sinus thrombosis (e.g. of the transverse or straight sinus) may be visible on plain CT or

MRI. CT venography should be considered if CT is undertaken first in any acute neurological presentation. MR venography should be included if MRI is undertaken and MRA is normal or the distribution of infarction is not typically arterial. On follow-up MRI small infarcts, which would otherwise be considered as SCI, may be documented.

Management

Infection and dehydration should be treated and seizures managed according to the appropriate protocol. There are no randomised trials in children or patients with SCD but in adults with venous sinus thrombosis in the general population, acute anticoagulation reduces mortality and there is some evidence for improvement in neurological outcome. Intravenous or treatment dose subcutaneous heparin should therefore be considered if the diagnosis is made in a patient with SCD.

Posterior Reversible Encephalopathy Syndrome

Posterior Reversible Encephalopathy Syndrome (PRES) is a severe acute neurological syndrome, encountered predominantly in children during the course of ACS. It is important to be aware to this complication, because incorrect management may result in avoidable morbidity and mortality.

Clinical Features

The typical presentation in the authors experience is of a child with a severe ACS who is fluid overloaded after excessive intravenous hydration and one or more simple blood transfusions. There is a notable increase in blood pressure, followed by an acute neurological deterioration with visual impairment, headache, seizure and sometimes transient weakness (which may be focal). It has also been reported after allogeneic bone marrow transplantation in children medicated with steroids and cyclosporin and during pregnancy.

Pathophysiology

The posterior circulation of the brain has a less well-developed compensatory autoregulation mechanism, and it is thought that microvascular integrity is impaired with the combination of vascular inflammation, endothelial damage, fluctuations in blood pressure and increased circulatory volume. This seems to result in edema, which is characteristically located in the white matter adjacent to the occipital and parietal cortices.

Investigations

Cerebral MRI imaging is needed to demonstrate white matter edema, and to exclude stroke. It is important to request T2 FLAIR and diffusion weighted imaging, as the white matter edema is visible on the former but there is no diffusion abnormality (Fig. 7.15).

Management

The patient should be managed on a high dependency unit with very careful monitoring of vital signs and neurological status. The main goals are to lower blood pressure gradually into the normal range, and to restore fluid balance. Rapid reduction of blood pressure may cause irreversible ischemia and parieto-occipital stroke. Anti-epileptic medication should be given to prevent further seizures. We have usually performed exchange transfusion with the aim of reducing HbS <30 %, even if there is no evidence of ischemia or vasculopathy. This will provide the optimal conditions for recovery from crisis and protect against secondary ischemic damage. Exchange transfusion must be performed with great care to ensure precise fluid balance and to prevent a rise in hemoglobin beyond 100 g/l.

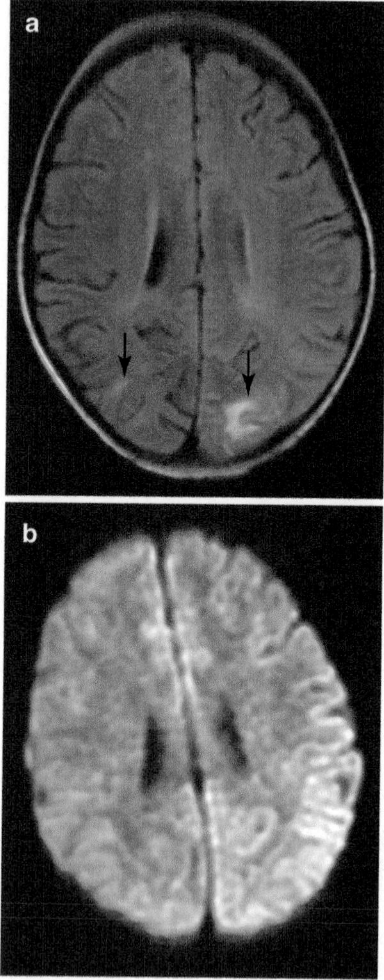

FIGURE 7.15 Cerebral MRI showing typical changes of posterior reversible encephalopathy syndrome (PRES). The child was age 5 and presented with severe acute chest syndrome, initially managed with 'hyper-hydration' and simple blood transfusion. Subsequently, he developed headache, hypertension, seizures and limb weakness. (**a**) T2 FLAIR showing abnormal high signal intensity in the subcortical white matter of the right and left occipital cortices (*arrows*) (**b**) Diffusion weighted imaging does not show enhancement in the occipital cortices, indicating that these lesions are not due to tissue infarction

Prognosis

After recovery, the prognosis is good. MRI should be repeated after 6–12 weeks to confirm resolution of abnormalities. We have experience of patients who have had recurrent episodes of PRES during subsequent severe crises, and although there may not be an indication for long-term transfusion, we would recommend that hydroxyurea is considered for long-term protection against severe vaso-occlusive crises which may precipitate further episodes of PRES.

Headaches

Headaches are common in children and adults with SCD, but there have been relatively few studies examining their causes and natural history. It is often not clear whether headaches are due to a significant underlying complication of SCD, or have a different explanation. The history may be helpful in identifying the cause. If they are most severe first thing in the morning this may suggest cerebral hemodynamic dysregulation related to obstructive sleep apnea or nocturnal hypoxemia- both common with SCD. Another common description is of troublesome headaches during the day while at school or work, and worse towards the end of the day. These may be related to chronic anemia, and are sometimes observed to reduce after enhancing hemoglobin level with hydroxyurea or regular blood transfusion.

Common causes of headaches in non-SCD patients should also be considered, including stress, eye-strain, and migraine. Headaches reported by adults with chronic pain symptoms are sometimes related to excessive use of opioid analgesics. Acute onset headache can be a feature of APC, but unusually severe headaches of sudden onset may indicate venous sinus thrombosis, intracerebral bleed or subarachnoid hemorrhage from aneurysmal bleeding, and patients should be instructed to attend urgently for assessment in this situation.

Investigations

Investigation of headache should include a detailed medical history to explore possible causes. Overnight sleep study should be performed in patients with morning headaches and symptoms of OSA. We recommend a low threshold for requesting cerebral MRI and MRA to investigate recurrent severe headaches interfering with normal functioning, in order to exclude cerebral ischemia, vasculopathy, and other intra-cerebral lesions.

Management

Patients with an abnormal sleep study or radiological findings of ischemia and/or vasculopathy should be treated according to findings. If other causes have been excluded, it may be appropriate to consider hydroxyurea treatment for patients with low hemoglobin and chronic headaches, which are interfering with normal activities. Where migraine is suspected, standard recommendations about excluding precipitants may be tried, together with standard treatment with simple analgesia or a triptan. A prophylactic agent such as propranolol may be necessary in patients with frequent migraine.

Bibliography

Adams RJ, McKie VC, Carl EM, et al. Long-term stroke risk in children with sickle cell diseasescreened with transcranial Doppler. Ann Neurol 1997;42:699–704.

Adams RJ, McKie VC, Hsu L, et al. Prevention of a first stroke by transfusion in children with sickle cell anemia and abnormal results on transcranial Doppler ultrasonography. N Engl J Med. 1998;339:5–11.

Adams FJ, Brambilla D, STOP 2 Trial Investigators. Discontinuing prophylactic transfusions used to prevent stroke in sickle cell disease. N Engl J Med. 2005;353:2769–78.

Bernandin F, Verlhac S, Arnaud C, et al. Impact of early transcranial Doppler screening and intensive therapy on cerebral vasculopathy outcome in a newborn sickle cell anemia cohort. Blood. 2011;117(4):1130–40.

DeBaun MR, Gordon M, McKinstry RC, et al. A Randomized Trial of Transfusion for Sickle Cell Anemia and Silent Cerebral Infarcts. New Engl J Med. 2014;371: 699–710.

Ganesan V, Kirkham F. Stroke and cerebrovascular disease in childhood. ICNA series of monographs in child neurology. London, UK: MacKeith Press; 2011.

Ohene-Frempong K, Weiner SJ, Sleeper LA, et al. Cerebrovascular accidents in sickle cell disease: rates and risk factors. Blood. 1998;91:288–94.

Ware R, Helms RW, SWiTCH Investigators. Stroke With Transfusions Changing to Hydroxyurea (SWiTCH). Blood. 2012;119(17): 3925–32.

Chapter 8
Renal and Urological Complications

Renal Dysfunction/Proteinuria

Pathophysiology

The kidney is susceptible to damage through several mechanisms which may work independently or in tandem. The disease process may effect glomerular and proximal tubular function as well as the urinary concentrating mechanism in the medulla. HbSS patients are generally the most severely affected, but significant pathology is also frequently observed in adults with HbSC, and even in carriers of SCD (**See** Chap. 1). A distal renal tubule concentrating defect is usually the first manifestation of renal damage, resulting in hyposthenuria (an inability to concentrate urine). Increased renal cortical blood flow due to anemia and high cardiac output is apparent from early childhood, and is associated with an increased glomerular filtration rate (GFR). Cortical and medullary ischaemia may also contribute to the increase in GFR. This glomerular hyperfiltration causes glomerular hypertrophy and is partly responsible for the progressive glomerular damage, which manifests initially as microalbuminuria and at later stages, proteinuria and progressive renal impairment. Histologically the glomeruli become enlarged and congested with sickled red cells, and there is proliferation

J. Howard, P. Telfer, *Sickle Cell Disease in Clinical Practice*, In Clinical Practice, DOI 10.1007/978-1-4471-2473-3_8,

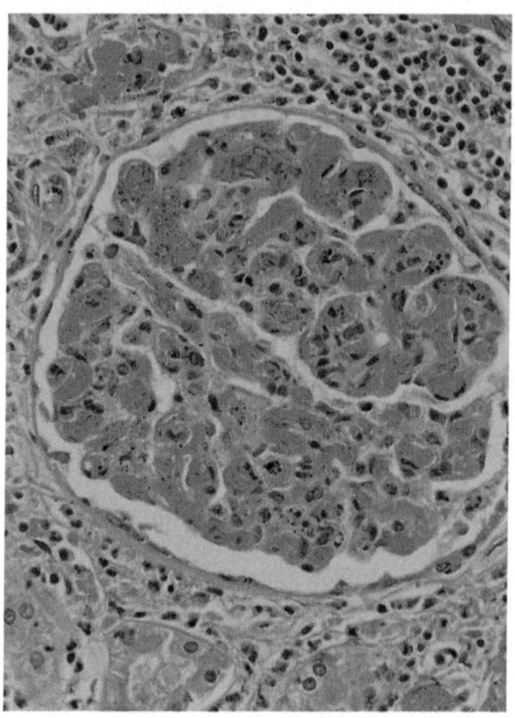

FIGURE 8.1 Renal biopsy showing an abnormal glomerulus which is enlarged with congested vessels and thickened mesangium

of the mesangium (Fig. 8.1). Later on the changes of focal and segmental glomerulosclerosis (FSGS) may develop.

In the medulla, there is occlusion of the vasa recta, (the vessels involved in the counter-current urinary concentration mechanism), together with ischemic damage and fibrosis. These changes are probably due to enhanced sickling in medullary conditions of slow blood flow, hemoconcentration, acidosis and low oxygenation.

In adults over the age of 30 there tends to be a progressive drop in GFR, and the insidious development of renal failure.

Prevalence

Microalbuminuria is present in up to 21 % of children and over 60 % of adults. The prevalence of proteinuria is around 4 % of children, 10 % of teenagers, 20 % of young adults and over 40 % in adults over 40 years of age. Renal insufficiency is seen in over 21 % of adults and progresses to end stage renal failure in 4-12 % of patients. It is likely that as survival and life expectancy improve, renal disease will become more common.

Clinical Presentation

Children who develop a concentrating defect pass large volumes of urine and often have problems with nocturnal enuresis, persisting into the teenage years. Adults may have nocturia, which can be associated with increasing proteinuria. Progressive loss of renal function occurs without noticeable symptoms and patients may present to clinic with end-stage renal failure.

Diagnosis and Screening

Screening and risk management for renal disease should be part of the routine care for children and adults and we recommend that these are part of the annual review. The assessment should include blood pressure monitoring, measurement of creatinine and eGFR and quantification of proteinuria by albumin-creatinine or protein-creatinine ratio (**See Chap.** 19). Children or their carers should be questioned about enuresis, hematuria and urinary infections.

Creatinine levels are usually low in SCD and a trend of increase over time, even if still within the normal range, may indicate worsening renal function. Patients presenting with proteinuria or chronic renal dysfunction should have investigations to rule out alternative causes including autoimmune disorders, chronic viral infection and structural abnormalities in the renal tract (demonstrable by ultrasound).

TABLE 8.1 Recommendations for screening and treatment of renal disease

Test result	Treatment option
Microalbuminuria (ACR >2.5 mg/mmol men, >3.5 mg/mmol women or PCR >15 mg/mmol)	No treatment but monitor regularly for progression
Proteinuria (ACR >30 mg/mmol or PCR >50 mg/mmol) which is persistent	Investigate for other causes of renal dysfunction. Commence ACEi or ARB and dose escalate if required
Hypertension >140/90 mmHg OR >130/80 mmHg if patient proteinuric	Treat with calcium antagonist or beta blocker as first line agent aiming for blood pressure of <130/80 mmHg (or <120/70 mmHg if proteinuric). ACEi may be a suitable alternative
Progressive anemia with renal impairment (Hb <65 g/l, reticulocytes <150 x109/l, eGFR <60 ml/min)	Trial of ESA. If ineffective after dose escalation, regular top-up transfusion may be required. Hemoglobin should not exceed 100 g/l

ACR Albumin Creatinine Ratio; *PCR* Protein Creatinine Ratio; *eGFR* estimated Glomerular Filtration Rate; *ACEi* Angiotensin Converting Enzyme inhibitor; *ARB* Angiotensin Receptor Blocker; *ESA* Erythropoiesis Stimulating Agent

Management

These patients should be reviewed by a renal physician with an interest in SCD, preferably in a specialist sickle-renal clinic. Renal biopsy should be considered, particularly in those with an atypical presentation or features which may suggest an alternative diagnosis. Recommendations for treatment are shown in Table 8.1.

Angiotensin-Converting Enzyme Inhibitors (ACEi)

These drugs act by inhibiting the Angiotensin II- mediated constriction of efferent glomerular arterioles, thereby decreasing the intra-glomerular pressure and glomerular permeability to albumin. The result is a decrease in proteinuria and normalization of glomerular filtration rate. This specific anti-proteinuric effect is combined with the action in controlling blood pressure. In diabetes mellitus, both ACEi and angiotensin receptor blockers (ARBs) have shown a similar anti-proteinuric effect and they have also been shown to slow the progression of renal impairment. There is some evidence that they also decrease proteinuria and microalbuminuria in patients with HbSS, and may also slow renal impairment. RCTs currently underway will help to define the role of these agents in managing renal impairment in SCD.

Hydroxyurea

The role of hydroxyurea in protecting against renal damage is not known. One of the primary endpoints of the BABYHUG trial was a reduction in GFR as measured by radionucleotide renal clearance. After 2 years of follow-up, GFR was increased to the same level in hydroxyurea and placebo groups. Although this result does not support hydroxyurea for routine use in preventing renal damage in early childhood, it does not rule out a potential role in longer-term control of renal disease in children and adults, and further controlled trials will be important to investigate this. Smaller case series suggest that hydroxyurea may be beneficial in selected patients. If it is to be used in those with established renal impairment, dose reduction is needed to avoid toxicity.

Blood Pressure Control

Blood pressure control is essential for patients with evidence of renal dysfunction. A target value of <130/80 is reasonable in adult patients who are proteinuric.

Erythropoiesis Stimulating Agents (ESAs)/Erythropoietin (EPO)

Although the majority of patients with SCD have high erythropoietin levels, the production of endogenous erythropoietin falls as GFR falls below 60 ml/min. ESAs may be useful in patients with a low GFR (<60 ml/min), anemia (Hb <65 g/l) and reticulocytopenia ($<150\times10^9$/l). A standard renal dose should be used with careful monitoring, aiming for a maximum hemoglobin level of 100 g/l. Iron replacement therapy (oral or parenteral) should be considered because of the high iron requirements of patients on ESAs, but should not be used if there is evidence of severe iron overload. High doses of ESAs are often needed, and patients who fail to respond at 4–8 weeks should have dose escalation. If they fail to respond to high levels of ESAs with adequate iron replacement there is probably little benefit in continuation. Even patients with a good response to ESAs may become transfusion dependent as their renal function worsens. Treatment could be continued in this situation if the ESA is shown to decrease transfusion requirements and prolong the interval between transfusions.

Blood Transfusion

There have been no long-term controlled studies to study whether regular transfusion prevents development and progression of renal disease. It is likely that correction of anemia and inhibition of sickling by transfusion of normal red cells will normalise GFR and reduce medullary sickling, but this needs to be formally evaluated. Chronic transfusion does have a role in managing progressive anemia in patients who do not respond to ESA's.

Pyelonephritis and Urinary Tract Infection (UTI)

UTI is common and is a potential cause of serious morbidity. This is not only because it can cause significant renal damage and contribute to progressive renal impairment, but also because infection often disseminates, leading to septicemia and systemic complications. Urinary tract infection is more common in women, especially during pregnancy and in those with an anatomical abnormality of the urinary tract. Infection is usually due to E.coli or other gram negative coliform organisms. Management of proven infection is with appropriate oral or intravenous antibiotics depending on the clinical scenario. It is important to request microbiological analysis of mid-stream urine sample in cases of unexplained fever or infective symptoms. Susceptible patients should be advised about standard measures to prevent UTI, and in some cases with recurrent UTI, it may be appropriate to recommend prophylactic antibiotics. These patients should be assessed jointly with a renal specialist or urologist.

Hematuria

Pathophysiology

Microscopic hematuria may be due to small microinfarcts in the kidney. Macroscopic hematuria is most commonly due to renal papillary necrosis secondary to medullary infarction, and if this leads to sloughing of the ischemic papilla it can cause severe hemorrhage and urinary tract obstruction. Renal papillary necrosis is also a rare complication seen in carriers if sickle cell. Other causes of hematuria not directly related to SCD include renal stones, and bladder tumours.

Incidence and Clinical Presentation

Renal papillary necrosis has been reported in up to 40–50 % of adult patients. In our experience, the usual presentation is with painless hematuria of sudden onset, and is fairly common in children with HbSS. There can be severe persisting bleeding and anemia.

Painless hematuria, especially in the over 40s may indicate malignant disease and needs urological referral.

Investigation

Initial blood tests include FBC, urea, electrolytes, creatinine, and coagulation screen. Renal USS may show evidence of calculi or of renal papillary necrosis but CT urography may be necessary to confirm the diagnosis. Painless hematuria in the over 40s needs urological referral for cystoscopy.

Treatment

Hematuria should initially be treated with fluids and blood transfusion if necessary. Urological input should be requested at an early stage, for consideration of bladder irrigation and surgical intervention. Occasionally desmopressin and antifibrinolytics have been used.

Medullary Carcinoma (MC)

This is a rare, aggressive cancer associated with SCD and also reported in carriers of sickle cell. The presentation is with abdominal pain and haematuria. MC is rapidly progressive and in some reports is metastatic at presentation. Prognosis is poor, as it is not usually sensitive to chemotherapy or radiotherapy.

Acute Renal Failure

Patients can present with acute renal failure (ARF) during an acute sickle crisis. One study reported an incidence of 2 % with acute painful crisis, and up to 14 % in severe ACS. Acute renal damage can be exacerbated by excessive use of non-steroidal anti-inflammatory drugs and nephrotoxic antibiotics. When an urgent transfusion or exchange transfusion is needed for an acutely unwell patient, this is occasionally complicated by a severe hemolytic or hyperhemolytic transfusion reaction with worsening of acute renal impairment (**See** Chap. 18).

Management of ARF in SCD requires specialist renal medicine input. Standard protocols used for ARF management are also appropriate for SCD. Renal ultrasound should be requested to exclude a post-renal cause. The principles of care include exclusion of reversible causes, maintenance of fluid balance, blood pressure control, good oxygenation, treatment of sepsis and renal replacement therapy as indicated. Hyperkalemia is more common in this patient group, probably due to renal tubular defects, and this needs careful monitoring and treatment. Urgent transfusion is needed if the hemoglobin is significantly below steady state level, and exchange transfusion should be undertaken if ARF is suspected to be due to multi-organ involvement with acute sickling.

End Stage Renal Failure (ESRF)

Renal replacement therapy for SCD is becoming common, reflecting the progressive deterioration in renal function seen in older patients. The options of hemodialysis, peritoneal dialysis or renal transplantation should be discussed as renal function deteriorates and before the patient becomes symptomatic with uremia, acidosis, fluid overload or hyperkalemia. It is advisable to start discussing options when eGFR decreases to around 20 ml/min. This will enable planning for arterio-venous fistula and preparation for renal transplantation. As patients develop ESRF, anemia often becomes more marked with a fall in hemoglobin of 10–20 g/l and it is worth considering a therapeutic trial of an ESA. Both haemodialysis and peritoneal dialysis can be considered. In our experience, there are advantages as well as significant morbidities associated with both approaches, and the choice will depend on individual factors.

Once on dialysis, patients with SCD have a poor prognosis, with a mean survival of only 4 years. They are also less likely to be placed on the transplant waiting list compared to other patient groups. Early transplantation (prior to commencing dialysis therapy) may be the best treatment option, and should be considered in patients with worsening renal function. Although outcomes from early studies were poor, these have improved so that patient and graft survival are now comparable with non-diabetic patients. Individuals with SCD who receive a renal transplant have a 7-year survival of 67 %, compared with a 10-year survival of only 14 % in those who remain on dialysis. Improved outcome is obtained with living donor rather than cadaveric donor transplants.

Exchange transfusion should be performed prior to transplantation to ensure HbS% of <30 % and should be continued at least in the immediate postoperative period. Hemoglobin levels often increase post-transplant and this may be accompanied by an increase in painful crisis and an increased stroke risk. Graft failure due to intra-renal sickling has also been described and long term exchange transfusion post-transplant to maintain HbS% <30% may be of benefit.

Priapism

Priapism is a painful, persistent, purposeless erection of the penis.

Prevalence

On direct questioning 35–89 % of men with SCD give a history of priapism. It is most common in adolescents and young adults, and the mean age at first episode is 15 years. Priapism can occur in any age and we have seen severe cases requiring surgical intervention in boys less than 5 years old. It is most common in HbSS, but is also frequent in adults with HbSC.

Pathophysiology

Priapism in SCD results from pooling of red cells in the corpora cavernosae. These are two distensible structures that surround the penile urethra and are anatomically separate from the glans penis. During normal erection, these structures fill with arterial blood, which pools and gradually deoxygenates until draining through penile veins at the resolution of the erection (Fig. 8.2). Clearly, this is not a good environment for HbS containing red cells and priapism results from sickling of red cells in the corpora cavernosae with vaso-occlusion of the drainage venules. A severe episode lasting more than 2 hours is likely to result in ischemia, inflammation and intra-cavernosal fibrosis with the end result of impotence.

Clinical Presentation

Priapism is often not recognized as a symptom of SCD, and young men may be embarrassed to talk about their symptoms.

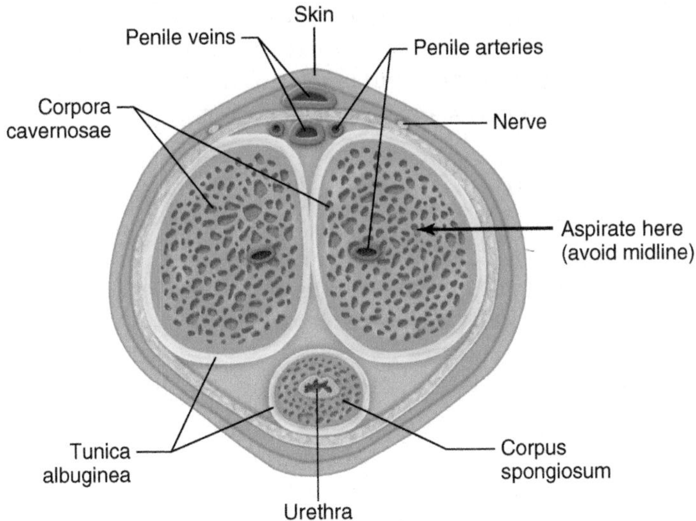

FIGURE 8.2 Cross section of shaft of penis showing site for aspiration

This typically results in late presentation to medical services. The onset is often at night, suggesting that nocturnal hypoxemia may have a role. Other precipitants include sexual activity, fever and intercurrent painful crisis. It is very useful to classify clinical presentations into two types.

Stuttering Priapism

This is self-limiting, lasting from a few minutes to an hour. Episodes usually occur at night and are often recurrent. These episodes are not thought to result in permanent penile damage or erectile dysfunction.

Fulminant Priapism

This is characterized by severe pain with a fully erect penis. Episodes last at least one hour and if not treated promptly, can result in permanent erectile dysfunction. Fulminant priapism should be treated as a medical emergency and patients should be instructed to seek urgent medical attention if an episode lasts for more than one to two hours. Fulminant priapism may occur de novo but about two thirds of episodes are preceded by a period of stuttering priapism.

Management

It is important to educate male patients and their parents about priapism from an early age, and this should be part of the general health advice given at annual review visits.

Self Treatment

Most patients report a variety of measures which seem to help to resolve an episode. These include exercise (press-ups seem particularly effective), hydration, a warm bath or shower and urination. Those with a previous history of priapism are generally prescribed an alpha adrenergic drug (see below) which can be taken to abort an episode if the above measures are ineffective. If priapism persists for more than one hour, urgent medical intervention is needed.

Urological Intervention

On arrival at hospital patients should be given fluids and analgesia: strong opioids are often needed. They should be catheterized if they have a palpable bladder. An alpha adrenergic drug (e.g. etilefrine) should be given if this has not been taken at home. Frequently, it is possible to resolve an episode by intra-cavernosal aspiration of 50–100 ml of blood. If initial aspiration is not successful this can be followed by intracavernosal injection of an alpha adrenergic agent (we recommend either phenylephrine in 200–500 μg aliquots, or etilefrine 5 mg) (Fig. 8.2). The procedure can be performed under local anaesthetic in the emergency department by a urologist. A penile block may be necessary, especially for a first episode. An arterial blood gas sample can be taken during aspiration and this will usually show low oxygenation typical of low-flow or stasis of blood. After this procedure, detumescence may be complete, partial or absent. In the latter case, a further aspiration under anaesthesia followed by a simple shunt procedure (a glans-corporal shunt) may be necessary. If this is not effective a definitive shunt insertion (a bilateral non-parallel spongiosum corporal shunt or a corporal-venous shunt) will be necessary, and this may require transfer to a specialist center.

We recommend a top up transfusion if the initial aspiration is not effective and if the hemoglobin is <65 g/l. Exchange transfusion should be done if the patient requires a shunt procedure or interventional surgery.

Secondary Prevention

Oral alpha adrenergic drugs are often helpful in controlling recurrent stuttering or fulminant episodes. In the authors' experience, the best option is long-acting etilefrine (Effortil) given at night (25–50 mg). Unfortunately this preparation is not currently available in the UK, and the short acting preparation (5–10 mg tds) is less effective. An alternative is ephedrine (15–30 mg). These drugs can potentially raise blood pressure and cause other adrenergic side effects so should only be commenced in patients with blood pressure of <140/90 and avoided in patients with ischemic heart disease, cardiac valvular stenosis or tachyarrythmias. We recommend monitoring blood pressure weekly for the first 2 weeks of therapy, monthly for the next 3 months and 2–3 monthly thereafter. It should be stopped if blood pressure exceeds 140/90 or if the patient develops palpitations. Their effect also decreases with prolonged use due to down-regulation of adrenergic receptors. Fortunately, stuttering priapism is often episodic, in periods lasting several days or weeks, and it is best to advise discontinuation once the episode has settled to enable the body to re-sensitize.

Diethylstiboestrol, has been used for prevention of priapism but has a high incidence of oestrogenic side effects. The phosphodiesterase type 5 (PDE5) inhibitors sildenafil and taldenafil have been effective in preventing stuttering priapism. These drugs should be used under urology supervision because they may precipitate priapism, and they should not be used to abort acute attacks. Their mechanism of action is probably via reconditioning of PDE5 regulatory function in the penis.

In the authors' experience, regular transfusion (usually exchange) is an effective means of controlling troublesome priapism if drug therapy is ineffective. Hydroxyurea may also be effective, but in some patients can make the situation worse so should be used with caution. The role of inhaled oxygen or positive airways pressure devices at night is unclear, but may be of value in patients with proven nocturnal hypoxia or obstructive sleep apnea.

Management of Erectile Dysfunction

Erectile dysfunction can be a long-term consequence of prolonged episodes of fulminant priapism. PDE5 inhibitors (e.g. sildenafil) can be used if there is a small amount of residual function, but care must be taken as they can precipitate priapism. Penile prostheses may be required to enable sexual function and in cases of severe priapism where there is a very high risk of erectile dysfunction they may be inserted acutely at the time of the shunt procedure.

Bibliography

Adeyoju AB, Olujohunbe ABK, Morris J, Yardumian A, Bareford D, et al. Priapism in SCD. Incidence, risk factors and complications. An international multi-center study. B J Urol. 2002;90:898–902.

Mantadakis E, Ewalt DH, Cavender JD, et al. Outpatient penile aspiration and epinephrine irrigation for young patients with sickle cell anemia and prolonged priapism. Blood. 2000;95:78–82.

Okafor UA, Aneke E. Outcome and challenges of kidney transplant in patients with sickle cell disease. J Transplant. 2013;2013:614610.

Sharpe CC, Thein SL. Sickle cell nephropathy – a practical approach. Br J Haematol. 2011;155:287–97.

Chapter 9
Bone and Joint Complications in Sickle Cell Disease

Avascular Necrosis

Chronic bone damage is one of the most important causes of long-term morbidity. Avascular necrosis (AVN) of the hip is a common complication in adults with HbSS and other genotypes of SCD. AVN of the hip, shoulder or spine results in chronic pain and loss of mobility and function.

Incidence

The incidence of asymptomatic disease is around 26 % in children and 41–80 % in young adults. Symptomatic disease is present in up to 50 % of adults. The hip is the most commonly affected joint followed by the shoulder and spine, and bilateral involvement is common.

Pathogenesis

Vaso-occlusion affecting the blood supply to the bone underlying the articular surfaces leads to ischemia and osteocyte necrosis. The ends of long bones (in particular the femur and humerus) are particularly susceptible to AVN, leading to a loss of structural integrity with eventual collapse of bone.

J. Howard, P. Telfer, *Sickle Cell Disease in Clinical Practice*, In Clinical Practice, DOI 10.1007/978-1-4471-2473-3_9,

Collapse of the articular surfaces is not reversible and leads to incongruity and severe joint damage. There is also a loss of adhesion between the bone and overlying articular cartilage, which can result in severe musculoskeletal pain.

Clinical Presentation

Patients usually present with increasing joint pain and stiffness. Symptoms may originate with an acute painful crisis which fails to settle. Mild groin pain on mobilization is a common early feature of hip AVN. Later, symptoms progress with pain at rest, night pain and eventually a painful immobile hip.

Asymptomatic shoulder AVN is also common and also tends to progress to a stiff, painful shoulder. The pain occurs initially on movement, but later patients develop rest pain. Although the rate of progression is slower than with hip AVN, one longitudinal study showed that over 80 % of patients had progressive disease during a mean follow-up of 20 years. In the same study over 60 % of patients with symptomatic shoulder disease required surgical intervention.

AVN is also commonly seen in the lumbosacral spine, resulting in back pain and stiffness.

Classification

There are several classifications used to monitor the progression of AVN which for clinical utility can be simplified into (i) precollapse and (ii) collapse. In pre-collapse, plain X-rays are normal or show sclerosis, however, bone infarction is apparent on MRI (Fig. 9.1). The development of subchondral fracture can be demonstrated on X-ray as the 'crescent sign'. In later stages, collapse is visible on plain X-ray with flattening of the femoral head, osteoarthritic changes and decreased joint space. The most advanced stage is complete joint destruction (Fig. 9.2).

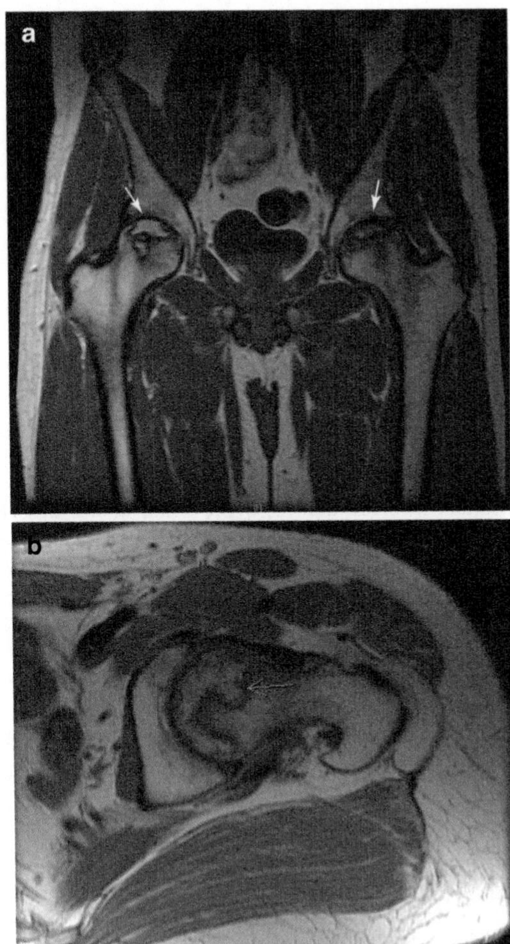

FIGURE 9.1 (**a**) MRI showing areas of avascular necrosis in both hips (*arrows*), but no evidence of collapse. This patient had bilateral hip pain, but hip X-Ray was normal. (**b**) MRI of the same patient showing an area of avascular necrosis without collapse (*arrow*)

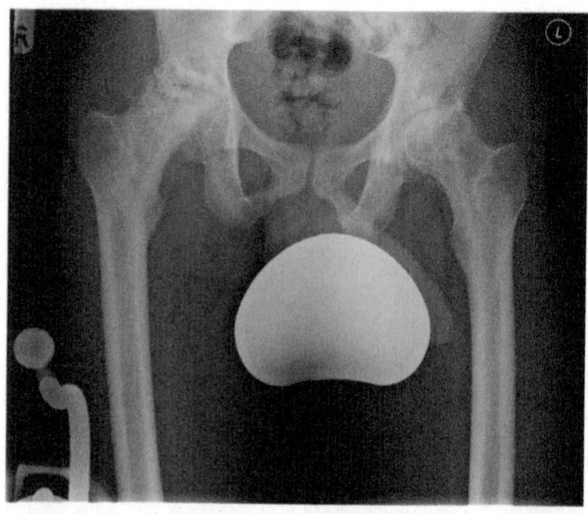

FIGURE 9.2 Bilateral advanced AVN. On the right side there is extrusion of the femoral head due to severe collapse and deformity. On the left there is a milder collapse, loss of joint space and a degenerative cyst in the roof of the acetabulum giving further indication of end-stage degeneration

Investigation

Plain X-Ray can be requested for initial investigation of patients presenting with chronic joint pain. If there is radiological evidence of AVN and collapse, no further radiological investigation is necessary. Xray may be normal in early disease and MRI may show the classical appearance of segmental collapse (Fig. 9.1), but may also show multiple small infarcts.

Management

Patients with AVN suffer from chronic musculoskeletal pain. An important goal of management is to develop an effective and acceptable analgesia regime, and this may require input from a chronic pain specialist.

Hip AVN: Early surgical intervention has not been shown to prevent progression, and screening of asymptomatic patients to identify early asymptomatic disease is not currently recommended. The only exception is in patients with AVN of one hip when it may be helpful to identify early AVN in the other. Patients with very early disease may benefit from non-weight-bearing exercise. Surgical core decompression of the hip has been advocated for AVN in other clinical settings, but was not shown to have any advantage over intensive physiotherapy in a randomised trial in SCD, and is not currently recommended as part of routine management for early AVN. It may be useful, however, in selected young patients with early disease (pre-collapse) and can reduce pain and prolong the time before hip replacement surgery is needed.

Once the hip has collapsed, a total hip replacement is usually needed and this should be performed in a center with experience in SCD. Early studies showed a high risk of prosthetic failure, with loosening of the implant and need for revision surgery. There were also high rates of surgical complications, including infection and intra-operative femoral fractures. These complications have reduced as specialist orthopaedic surgeons become more experienced in operating on SCD patients and with use of modern techniques and implants. The best contemporary outcomes have been obtained using cementless ceramic-on-ceramic implants. In one of our centers, the current failure rate is <5 % at 7.5 years.

Shoulder AVN: Early stage disease can be treated with analgesia and physiotherapy, although arthroscopy and decompression may be of benefit. End stage disease requires shoulder hemiarthroplasty. Fewer cases of shoulder AVN need implant surgery because the shoulder is not a weight bearing joint and collapse is less commonly seen.

AVN in Children

Children are also at risk of AVN. We have observed hip AVN fairly commonly, predominantly in pre-pubertal teenagers with HbSS, but also occasionally with HbSC. Radiological changes are similar to those seen in adults, but with an unfused epiphysis. The immaturity of the growth plate suggests that some regrowth and remodelling of the femoral head may be possible prior to epiphyseal fusion, provided the femoral head is not collapsed.

Some of the children with severe AVN had been taking hydroxyurea for control of acute crises. In these cases, our policy has been to switch treatment to regular transfusions, with the aim of improving perfusion of the femoral head to aid in healing. This is combined with reduction in weight bearing and physiotherapy. Most of these children have done well, with good symptomatic improvement, and in some cases, evidence of radiological improvement.

Hip replacement surgery is not advised in children unless there is irreversible severe damage, deformity and severe symptoms which do not respond to conservative treatment. The silent infarct transfusion (SIT) trial results have recently been published, and show a significant reduction in the incidence of hip AVN in children with silent cerebral ischaemia who were transfused over a 3 year period, compared to those in the observation arm. This is an important observation, but as yet it is unclear how to translate the finding into clinical practice.

Bone and Joint Infection

Incidence

Osteomyelitis is an important and common complication of SCD, but septic arthritis less so. A review of 2000 admissions of adults with SCD shown that 7 % were due to osteomylitis and 0.3 % to septic arthritis.

Pathophysiology

In developed countries, salmonella is the commonest cause of bone infection in SCD, particularly non-typical serotypes such as typhimurium, enteritidis and paratyphi B. It is thought that the origin of these infections is through ingestion of contaminated food, followed by hematogenous dissemination of bacteria to areas of bone that have become necrotic. Staphylococcus aureus osteomyelitis is reported, but much less commonly, and other gram-negative enteric bacteria are also occasionally isolated. Septic arthritis can be associated with osteomyelitis at a distant site.

Clinical Presentation

Osteomyelitis presents with local pain and tenderness, warmth, swelling and fever. An acute painful crisis usually presents with similar features, and differentiation can be very difficult. It is important to avoid unnecessary surgical intervention, but also not to miss the diagnosis of osteomyelitis because of the risk of progressive bone or joint damage. The femur, tibia and humerus are the sites most commonly affected.

Diagnosis

Osteomyelitis should be suspected in a patient with local pain, bony tenderness and swelling associated with a high swinging fever, and which fails to resolve over the typical time course of an acute painful crisis. These features are not incompatible with an acute painful crisis with severe bone infarction, where pain, swelling and fever can also persist for many days. In osteomyelitis white blood cell count and C-reactive protein are usually significantly elevated. Blood cultures, if positive, are helpful in confirming the diagnosis and guiding antibiotic choice.

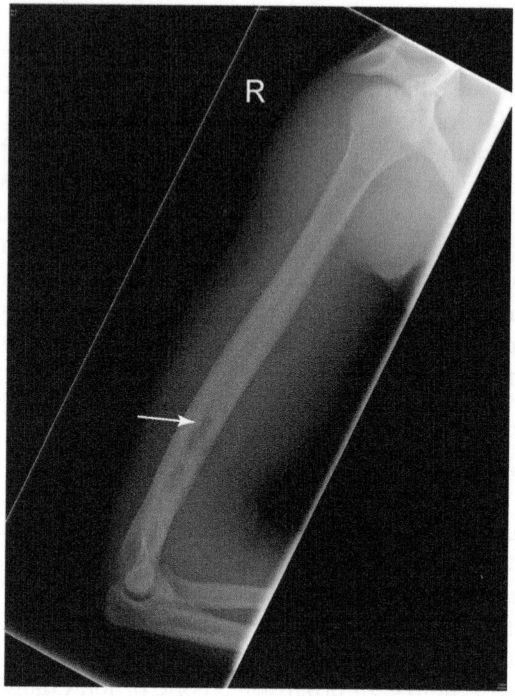

FIGURE 9.3 Plain radiographs showing area of chronic osteomyelitis in right humerus (*arrow*)

Plain X-Rays are normal in the early stages of infection, but characteristic changes can be seen in chronic osteomyelitis (Fig. 9.3). Ultrasound can be helpful in the hands of experienced radiologists and the finding of increased sub-periosteal fluid of over 4 mm has been reported to be useful in differentiating osteomyelitis from bone infarction. MRI scanning with gadolinium enhancement demonstrates bone oedema secondary to infection and can be helpful in diagnosis, but bone infarction can also cause marrow oedema, giving a similar appearance. MRI scanning may also be useful in following up response to treatment. Bone scans and radiolabelled leucocyte scans do not differentiate between infection and infarction. Bone aspiration or biopsy and drainage can be a useful diagnostic investigation as well as an important part of surgical treatment but cultures are often negative once antibiotics have been started. It is worthwhile requesting bacterial genome testing (16s ribosomal DNA) on bone aspiration samples. In our experience this has enabled identification of the underlying pathogen when cultures are negative.

Treatment

Initial empiric treatment with intravenous antibiotics should cover Salmonella, staphylococcus aureus and gram-negative enteric organisms until culture and sensitivity results are available. Antibiotics active against salmonella include ceftriaxone, a third generation cephalosporin, and ciprofloxacin which can also be given orally. In order to eradicate bone infection, antibiotics need to be continued for at least 6 weeks, and in some cases 3 months or more. Orthopedic and microbiology input is needed to plan treatment and to ensure long-term eradication. Surgical drainage may be necessary when there is an intraosseous collection of pus or sequestrum.

Vitamin D Deficiency

Vitamin D promotes intestinal absorption of calcium and functions in concert with parathyroid hormone and calcitonin to maintain blood calcium levels and normal bone mineral content. Vitamin D is present in oily fish, and fortified foods, but is otherwise relatively sparse in the normal diet. The main source of Vitamin D is biosynthesis from 7-dehydrocholesterol by the action of ultaviolet radiation on the skin. It is sequentially converted into 25-hydroxy Vitamin D (25-OHD) and 1,25 dihydroxy Vitamin D, the latter being metabolically active.

Deficiency can result in hypocalcaemia, depletion of skeletal calcium and bone damage. In children, severe vitamin D deficiency can result in hypocalcaemic seizures and rickets, while the elderly develop osteomalacia. Vitamin D status is commonly assessed by 25-OHD levels. There is some variability in advice about levels associated with biochemical deficiency and further confusion due to use of different units in the USA (ng/ml) and other countries (nmol/l). It is generally accepted that serum levels of 20ng/ml (50nmol/l) are required for bone health, and a level below 10ng/ml (25 nmol/l) is often described as severe deficiency.

Incidence

Vitamin D deficiency is common in SCD patients, occurring in up to 75–80 % of those studied, more commonly in adults than children. This high prevalence is probably due to a combination of inadequate synthesis in pigmented skin, reduced exposure to sunlight, poor diet and chronic ill health. Low bone mineral density (BMD) is also common and has been shown in 40–80 % of patients with SCD in some studies.

Pathophysiology

Patients with SCD may have bone defects due to chronic hemolysis, marrow expansion, osteonecrosis and bony infarction. The interaction of these abnormalities with Vitamin D deficiency may contribute to poor bone health. Low Vitamin D levels can be associated with increased risk of low BMD, but this is not invariable.

Clinical Picture

In the general population there is increasing evidence that Vitamin D deficiency may be associated with chronic musculoskeletal pain and fatigue. The association of Vitamin D deficiency and chronic pain and fatigue in SCD has not yet been fully elucidated, but it is likely that Vitamin D deficiency plays a role in some cases.

Screening and Treatment

We recommend assessment of Vitamin D (25 OHD) levels at least annually. Bone density assessment may be indicated if there is a clinical suspicion of osteoporosis, but it is not a routine part of the annual assessment in SCD. If patients are found to be Vitamin D deficient they should be treated with Calcium and Vitamin D supplementation according to local protocols. A pilot study has shown fewer pain days and improved quality of life in children and adolescents treated with high dose Vitamin D, irrespective of baseline vitamin D level, but this needs further prospective study.

Bibliography

Al Omran A. Multiple drilling compared with standard core decompression for avascular necrosis of the femoral head in sickle cell disease patients. Arch Orthop Trauma Surg. 2013;133(5):609–13.

Almeida A, Roberts I. Bone involvement in sickle cell disease. B J Haematol. 2005;129(4):482–90.

Goodman BM, Artz N, Radford B, Chen I. Prevalence of vitamin D deficiency in adults with sickle cell disease. J Natl Med Assoc. 2010;102:332–5.

Hernigou P, Habibi A, Bachir D, Galacteros F. The natural history of asymptomatic osteonecrosis of the femoral head in adults with sickle cell disease. J Bone Joint Surg Am. 2006;88:2565–72.

Hernigou P, Daltro G, Flouza-Lachaniette CH, Roussignol X, Poignard A. Septic arthritis in adults with sickle cell disease often is associated with osteomyelitis or osteonecrosis. Clin Orthop Relat Res. 2010;468(6):1676–81.

Issa K, Naziri Q, Maheshwari A, Rasquinha V, Delanois R, Mont M. Excellent results and minimal complications of total hip arthroplasty in sickle cell hemoglobinopathy at mid-term follow-up using cementless prosthetic components. J Arthroplasty. 2013;28:(9):1693–8.

Neumayr F, Aguilar C, Earles A, Jergesen H, Haberkern C, Kammen B, Nancarrow P, Padua E, Milet M, et al. Physical therapy alone compared with core decompression and physical therapy for femoral head osteonecrosis in sickle cell disease. Results of a multicenter study at a mean of three years after treatment. J Bone Joint Surg Am. 2006;88:2573–82.

Osunkwo I, Ziegler TR, McCracken C, et al. High dose vitamin D therapy for chronic pain in children and adolescents with sickle cell disease: results of a randomized double blind pilot study. B J Haematol. 2012;159(2):211–5.

Poignard A, Flouzat-Lachaniette C, Amzelleg J, Galacteros F, Hernigou P. The natural progression of symptomatic humeral head osteonecrosis in adults with sickle cell disease. J Bone Joint Surg Am. 2012;94(2):156–62.

Chapter 10 Ophthalmological Complications

Introduction

The conjunctiva, anterior segment, retina, retinal vessels, choroid and optic nerve are all susceptible to damage due to the effects of SCD, with the possible consequences of transient or permanent visual impairment.

Proliferative and Non-proliferative Retinopathy

Definitions

Retinopathy is the most common opthalmological complication seen in SCD. It is classified into two subtypes.

Non-proliferative retinopathy (NPR) is common, but does not lead to visual loss and does not need intervention. Features on retinoscopy include salmon patches (intra-retinal hemorrhage) schisis cavities (retinal deficits left after resolution of intraretinal hemorrhage), iridescent spots, black sunbursts (choroidoretinal scars from pigmentation around vessels), angioid streaks (breaks in Bruch's membrane) or macular remodelling.

J. Howard, P. Telfer, *Sickle Cell Disease in Clinical Practice*, In Clinical Practice, DOI 10.1007/978-1-4471-2473-3_10,

Proliferative Retinopathy (PR) The progressive clinical features are described in the Goldberg staging scheme (Table 10.1).

Pathophysiology

Retinopathy is due to vaso-occlusion of the retinal vessels. The arteriolar occlusion and subsequent loss of capillary perfusion leads to ischemia, and release of growth factors which stimulate new vessel formation (neovascularization). These fragile new vessels grow out from the surface of the retina and have a tendency to bleed (vitreous hemorrhage). Intraocular blood is degraded, but repeated hemorrhage leads to fibrous tissue accumulation which contracts and pulls on the underlying retina resulting in retinal holes and detachment. There is a balance between pigment epithelium-derived factor (PEDF) which is anti-angiogenic, and vascular endothelial growth factor (VEGF). An increase of VEGF relative to PEDF is associated with neovascularization.

Table 10.1 Goldberg staging scheme for proliferative retinopathy

Stage	**Clinical Findings**
Stage I: Peripheral arteriolar occlusions	Early stages of vaso-occlusion. Vessels are initially dark red but later become 'silver wires'
Stage II: Vascular remodelling, formation of arteriovenous anastomoses	Blood diverted from occluded to adjacent vessels
Stage III: Peripheral retinal neovascularization	'Sea fan' formation- neovascular tufts. These can grow and gain fibrous envelopes (elevated ridges)
Stage IV: Vitreous hemorrhage	
Stage V: Retinal detachment	The fibrous sea fans and residual organised blood clot from vitreous haemorrhage pull on the retina leading to detachment.

Prevalence

PR is more common in HbSC than HbSS, (prevalence rates of in 8.4 % for HbSS and 39 % for HbSC). It is most common in the 20–39 year age group but can occur in any age and is seen earlier in patients with HbSC than other genotypes.

Clinical Features

The majority of PR is asymptomatic. Stages I to III are usually identified on screening, are not associated with visual loss and resolve spontaneously in 20–60 % of cases. The usual presentation of vitreous hemorrhage is with acute, transient visual disturbance, often described as 'floaters' in the eye. Acute sight-threatening visual loss, which patients often describe as 'a curtain coming down' or as the development of a 'shadow' across the visual field can be seen with retinal detachment but is also a feature of retinal artery occlusion. Patients with these symptoms should be urgently reviewed by an ophthalmologist. Visual loss due to hemorrhage may improve over time as the hemorrhage is reabsorbed, but the patient may be left with diminished visual acuity in the affected eye.

Management

Enquiry about visual symptoms and education about the risk of visual complications of SCD should be part of the routine outpatient review in children and adults with all SCD genotypes. Patients should be aware that they need to attend urgently for assessment if presenting with acute deterioration in vision. Vitreous hemorrhage and retinal detachment may require surgical intervention, either immediately or, more commonly, when the hemorrhage has settled. Advances in vitreoretinal surgical techniques allow safer surgery with fewer complications than have been reported in older series. There are anecdotal reports of anti-VEGF antibodies (Bevacizumab) causing regression of retinal neovascularization in SCD, but this needs further investigation in clinical trials.

Prevention

Panretinal photocoagulation laser treatment can be used to prevent complications of PR, but may cause unnecessary retinal damage. Improvements in laser treatment have lead to decreased complications so that photocoagulation may now have a greater role in patients with bilateral proliferative disease, spontaneous hemorrhage, rapid growth of neovascular tissue or when vision in the other eye has been lost. Regular retinal screening is not required for asymptomatic children, and in view of the slow progressive nature of PR and the high incidence of spontaneous regression is probably not of benefit for asymptomatic adults. A pragmatic approach is to screen patients once as a baseline and if there is no evidence of PR offer further screening only if symptoms develop. Patients with PR should be offered regular screening and furthermore, patients with visual loss in one eye should have regular screening of the other eye. Patients should be informed about the risks of ophthalmic complications and instructed to attend urgently if they develop visual symptoms.

New imaging techniques, such as Ocular Coherence Tomography, microperimetry and scanning laser ophthalmoscopes, with wider fields of vision and better resolution can identify early retinal changes and temporal thinning in asymptomatic patients, but their role in screening in SCD is not yet clear.

Central Retinal Artery Occlusion

Central retinal artery or segmental retinal artery occlusion is an important cause of acute uni-ocular visual loss which tends to affect adolescents and young adults with HbSS, and

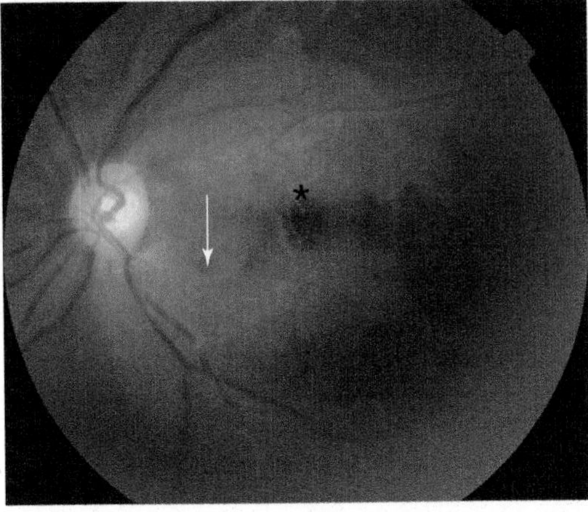

FIGURE 10.1 Occlusion of cilio-retinal artery in a child with HbSS (*arrow*). The cherry-red spot at the macula, typical of retinal artery occlusion in white people, appears black in this population (*asterisk*)

occurs either spontaneously or during the course of an acute vaso-occlusive crisis. Patients usually present with an acute visual loss (often described as a 'curtain coming down'). Occlusion of a branch retinal artery will cause an acute loss of a segment of the visual field of the affected eye. The characteristic ophthalmological features are retinal pallor, visible absence of the affected artery, and sometimes a cherry red spot at the macula (Fig. 10.1). The spot is actually black when it affects those with black skin pigmentation. There is no means of predicting this complication. Furthermore, although these patients are often anti-coagulated or treated with urgent exchange transfusion, there is no evidence that any intervention can prevent retinal infarction.

Other Causes of Visual Loss

Anterior segment ischemia and secondary glaucoma are also associated with visual loss in the SCD population.

In our experience, the commonest visual defects in children are field deficiencies due to cerebral damage with acute ischemic stroke. We have also had cases of ophthalmic artery occlusion secondary to occlusion of the extracerebral Internal Carotid artery.

Blunt trauma to the eye can cause a hyphema (blood settling in the anterior chamber of the eye). High intra-ocular pressure can result and patients are particularly at risk of optic nerve damage as a result. It is essential that patients with hyphemas are assessed for sickle cell disease and the intra-ocular pressures are monitored carefully, otherwise irreversible visual loss may result.

Bibliography

Downes SM, Hambleton IR, Chuang EL, Lois N, Serjeant GR, Bird AC. Incidence and natural history of proliferative sickle cell retinopathy: observations from a cohort study. Ophthalmology. 2005;112(11):1869–75.

Fox PD, Vessey SJR, Forshaw ML, Serjeant GR. Influence of genotype on the natural history of untreated proliferative sickle retinopathy an angiographic study. Br J Ophthalmol. 1991;75:229–31.

Williamson TH, Rajput R, Laidlaw DAH, Mokete B. Vitreoretinal management of the complications of sickle cell retinopathy by observation or pars plana vitrectomy. Eye. 2009;23(6):1314–20.

Chapter 11
The Spleen

Introduction

The pathophysiology of splenic damage is described in Chap. 1. Loss of splenic function can be demonstrated as early as three months of age in HbSS. On routine examination in the out-patient clinic, the spleen often enlarges sufficiently to become palpable between 6 and 18 months of age, and thereafter becomes inpalpable, atrophic and non-functional by the age of 3–5 years (Fig. 11.1). Even if the spleen continues to be palpable, or appears to be of normal size on ultrasound scan, it is likely to be hypofunctional, and we recommend that the national guidelines for protection against infection for asplenic patients should be followed for all SCD patients (See Chap. 12).

Acute Splenic Sequestration

Acute splenic sequestration (ASS) is an important and potentially life-threatening complication seen most commonly in infants with HbSS. It is caused by the trapping (sequestering) of a large volume of red cells in the spleen, leading to splenic enlargement and rapidly progressive anemia (See Fig. 1.5).

J. Howard, P. Telfer, *Sickle Cell Disease in Clinical Practice*,
In Clinical Practice, DOI 10.1007/978-1-4471-2473-3_11,

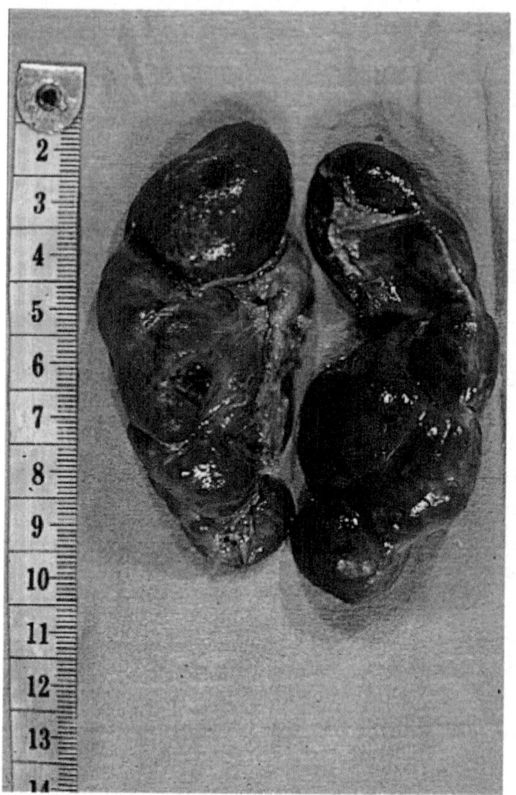

FIGURE 11.1 Shrunken involuted spleen

Definition

The definition used in the Cooperative Study of Sickle Cell Disease is a fall in hemoglobin level of least 20 % associated with enlargement of the spleen by at least 2 cm from steady state. This emphasizes the need for information on steady state values, which should be documented at the child's annual review visit.

Prevalence

The highest incidence rate is seen in HbSS children during the age range 3 months to 2 years. The majority of episodes occur before the age of 5 years. The overall rate in childhood is about 12 %. In HbSC, episodes are generally seen in children age 5 years and over, and the overall rate in childhood is about 6 %.

ASS is also seen in older children or in adults with milder genotypes, but generally without such severe sequelae.

Clinical Presentation

Patients usually present with abdominal discomfort, lethargy and increasing splenomegaly. ASS may progress rapidly, with a precipitous drop in the hemoglobin level and circulatory collapse. Over 50 % of cases have an associated fever, infection or painful crisis. The anaemia is usually accompanied by a pronounced reticulocytosis. Historical mortality rates are as high as 44 %, but with modern management are less than 1 %. The clinical features of ASS were well described in a cohort of Jamaican children with HbSS. The authors identified a less severe presentation which they described as a 'minor' episode of ASS, defined as a drop of 20 g/l in hemoglobin together with evidence of an active bone marrow (increased reticulocyte count) and an acutely enlarging spleen. They differentiate this from a major episode, where these features were associated with circulatory collapse. These minor episodes appeared to be predictive of acute life threatening episodes. They noted a variety of non-specific symptoms associated with minor episodes, and in some cases the patient had no symptoms at all. This description is very typical of what is observed in our clinical practice. It is important to correctly diagnose these episodes, as they can easily be missed. They also described some patients who developed hypersplenism (which they defined as a chronic enlargement of the spleen, with a persistent fall in haemoglobin of at least 20 g/l and a low platelet count). They noted that episodes of ASS associated with hypersplenism in young children also carried a poor prognosis and an increased risk of mortality. Older children may have a more benign presentation with gradual splenic enlargement and slowly progressive anemia.

Management

Parents should be instructed about ASS and palpation of the abdomen from 3 months of age, so that severe episodes can be anticipated and dealt with quickly. Suspicion of ASS should trigger immediate hospital referral. This early warning mechanism only works if the acute medical staff understand the acute care pathway to be followed if the parent believes the spleen is getting large, and pediatricians should be aware of the rapidly progressive nature of this condition and its high associated mortality. A common situation occurs when the infant already has an enlarged spleen, and there is moderate increase in size associated with a drop from an already low hemoglobin level. This is more confusing for the parent in deciding when and if to bring their child in for assessment. This is a potentially serious situation and should be diagnosed as a significant episode of ASS.

Acute episodes resolve rapidly with simple top-up transfusion of 10–15 ml/kg red cells aiming to return the hemoglobin to the patient's baseline level (without aiming for a particular percentage of HbS). It is important not to over-transfuse (Hb >110 g/l), as this can result in circulatory overload and increased blood viscosity. Sequestered red cells can re-enter the circulation as the sequestration resolves leading to a further increase in hemoglobin level, so there should be ongoing monitoring of hemoglobin levels as the patient recovers. Exchange transfusion would only be indicated after an initial top-up transfusion if there were additional complications such as acute chest syndrome or stroke.

In over 50 % of cases, episodes of ASS are recurrent, and there may be a tendency to increasing severity over time. Splenectomy is generally indicated for recurrent events, however, it is important to consider this option carefully. Although the spleen is hypofunctional in SCD, in many children there is residual function, and removal of the spleen in childhood will increase the vulnerability to bacterial infection and malaria (important for those who are going on holiday or at risk of being deported back to Africa). Splenectomy should not be undertaken for a single episode of ASS, and for very young children who are having recurrent episodes, an alternative approach of regular transfusion until the age of 5 is effective in controlling ASS. At this age the risks of ASS are less, and the child can be more safely reassessed off transfusion.

Splenic sequestration may be followed by transient hypersplenism or chronic splenic enlargement.

Chronic Splenomegaly

Splenic function is better preserved in patients with a milder phenotype. This includes some HbSS patients with co-inheritance of alpha thalassemia, or with high persisting HbF levels, and the genotypes HbSC and HbS β^{+} thalassemia. These patients often develop splenomegaly later in childhood, persisting into adult life. Complications of chronic hypersplenism, include thrombocytopenia, low or decreasing steady state hemoglobin level and a hypermetabolic state. Chronic splenomegaly also contributes to growth retardation and delayed puberty. Such patients may have recurrent acute episodes of splenic infarction (severe pain in the left upper quadrant with a tender, enlarged spleen) in later life. Chronic splenomegaly and its complications need to be carefully monitored on routine clinic visits.

If there is evidence of progressive enlargement with clinical features of hypersplenism and/or recurrent episodes of crisis with splenic sequestration, splenectomy may be indicated. In older children, the clinical benefits are often notable, with a significant improvement in energy levels, a rise in steady state hemoglobin and acceleration in growth.

Post-splenectomy Care

Long-term prophylaxis for asplenia is strongly recommended for patients after splenectomy. It is important to remind splenectomised patients about the risks of infection regularly and to check on compliance with penicillin and vaccination status at the annual review visit.

Bibliography

Brousse V, et al. Acute splenic sequestration crisis in sickle cell disease. Br J Hematol. 2012;156:643–8.

Topley JM, et al. Acute splenic sequestration and hypersplenism in the first five years in homozygous sickle cell disease. Archives of Disease in Childhood. 1981;56:765–9.

Chapter 12
Infection and Infection Prophylaxis

Introduction

Infection is an important cause of morbidity and mortality in SCD. This is partly due to loss of the normal protective function of the spleen, which contributes to the control of invasive infection by removing foreign particles and damaged blood cells from the circulation. Splenic function is also necessary for generating a normal immunoglobulin response to some infections. Hyposplenia in infants is associated with a deficiency in the IgM response to encapsulated bacteria which further increases the risk of invasive infection. *Streptococcus pneumoniae*, *Neisseria meningitides*, *Hemophilus influenzae* type b, salmonella species and gram negative enteric organisms can all cause serious systemic infection. Prior to the introduction of pneumococcal prophylaxis, invasive pneumococcal disease (IPD) was the most common cause of death in SCD. Infection can progress rapidly causing shock, disseminated intravascular coagulation and adrenal hemorrhage. Children below the age of 2 with HbSS are at highest risk of overwhelming IPD.

There is also an increased risk of gram negative bacterial infection affecting the urinary tract and biliary system, as well as non-typhi salmonella infection causing generalized sepsis and osteomyelitis. These are described in more detail in the Chapters 8, 9 and 12 which cover the relevant organs and

J. Howard, P. Telfer, *Sickle Cell Disease in Clinical Practice*, In Clinical Practice, DOI 10.1007/978-1-4471-2473-3_12,

systems. Acute chest syndrome and other acute vaso-occlusive crises can be provoked by viral infections of the respiratory tract and 'atypical' organisms such as *Mycoplasma pneumoniae* and *Chlamydia pneumoniae.*

Malaria

Carriers of sickle cell (HbAS) are protected against severe, life-threatening falciparum malaria because intra-erythrocytic HbS impairs parasitic invasion of erythrocytes, inhibits multiplication of parasites and enhances parasitic clearance in the spleen. This resistance to malaria is not apparent in HbSS or other sickle genotypes, and malarial infection in SCD is associated with increased mortality and morbidity. In malarial-endemic countries, children with SCD who present with severe anemia may have co-existent malaria. Long-term malarial prophylaxis has been shown to decrease the rate of severe anemia, sickle crises and to reduce mortality. Patients with SCD travelling to countries where there is a risk of malaria should be advised to take anti-malarial prophylaxis following the current standard recommendations for drug therapy applicable to the part of the world where they are travelling.

Invasive Pneumococcal Disease (IPD)

Pneumococcus is another name for the bacterium *Streptococcus pneumoniae.* The infections included in the term IPD are pneumonia, meningitis and septicaemia. Another common site for pneumococcal infection is the middle ear (otitis media), though this is not classified as IPD. Asymptomatic carriage of pneumococcus in the throat and nasopharynx is common in infants, but does not usually result in IPD. It is important to make a definitive microbiological diagnosis of pneumococcal infection, but this can be difficult in practice. Sputum is often unobtainable in the early stages

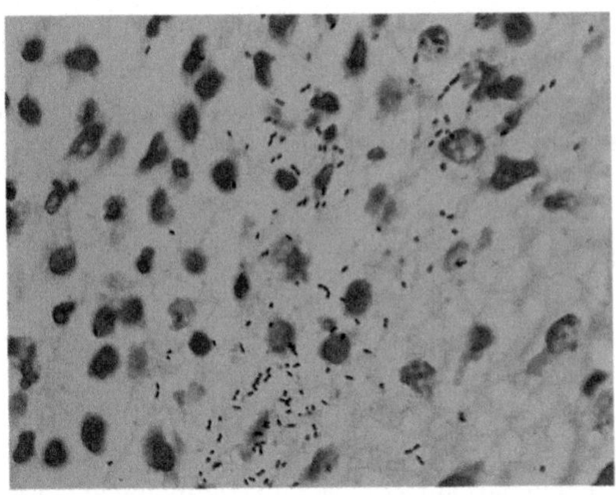

FIGURE 12.1 Postmortem sample of meningeal tissue from a patient with pneumococcal meningitis. Smear shows gram-positive diplococci

of pneumococcal pneumonia, and it is challenging to obtain positive cultures from sputum, blood or cerebrospinal fluid because of the need for special culture conditions and meticulous laboratory technique. Sometimes the infection is diagnosed on post-mortem tissue by gram stain (Figure 12.1). Other microbiological techniques include assay for urinary pneumococcal antigen (which is not specific to IPD and may also be positive with nasopharyngeal carriage in infants) and bacterial 16s ribosomal DNA analysis of samples from otherwise sterile sites, including cerebrospinal fluid.

Successful treatment of IPD requires supportive care and immediate administration of high dose intravenous antibiotics active against pneumococcus. Standard local guidelines for treating IPD should be followed, and the patient should be monitored very carefully for additional acute complications of SCD which may require specific intervention as described elsewhere in this book.

Before pneumococcal prophylaxis was introduced in the USA, the rate of IPD in infants was about 10 episodes per 100 patient years of follow-up. IPD was a major cause of childhood death in the Jamaican Sickle Cell Cohort Study and the Infant Cohort of the Cooperative Study of SCD in USA. These studies recruited before oral penicillin prophylaxis was given routinely.

Penicillin Prophylaxis

A randomized controlled trial in the early 1980s showed that prophylaxis with oral penicillin in children <3 years of age decreased the risk of invasive pneumococcal disease (IPD) by 84 %. This led to a recommendation for oral penicillin prophylaxis starting at 3 months of age and continuing at least until the age of 5 years. Those with a history of IPD were recommended to continue oral penicillin in the longer term. Whether penicillin prophylaxis should be continued in older children and adults is controversial. A US trial showed no significant increase of pneumococcal infection if penicillin V prophylaxis was stopped at 5 years. This was a relatively small trial with a low incidence of infections in both treatment and observation arms, and of itself, does not provide sufficient evidence to justify stopping penicillin. Although the incidence of IPD is reduced after the age of 5 years, most reports have shown that IPD is still a significant cause of morbidity and mortality in older children and adults.

British guidelines suggest penicillin prophylaxis should used for hyposplenic patients at highest risk of IPD. This includes those less than 16 years and above 50 years, those with inadequate serological response to pneumococcal vaccination or a history of invasive pneumococcal disease. Patients not categorized at high risk, or who are reluctant to take long-term antibiotics should be counselled about the risks and benefits of lifelong antibiotics. Patients who choose to discontinue prophylaxis should be vaccinated appropriately, and should be given a supply of appropriate antibiotics which should be taken if they develop signs or symptoms of infection. They should also be advised to seek medical attention at an early stage if the infection is severe and/or not responding to initial home management.

Vaccination

Vaccination schedules are frequently updated and whilst the information below is correct at the time of going to press, the latest Department of Health advice should be reviewed.

Pneumococcal Vaccination

Polysaccharide pneumococcal vaccine (PPV) was introduced in the 1980s, and the current 23-valent vaccine (Pneumovax®) in combination with oral penicillin, appears to be effective in controlling IPD. Pneumovax is poorly immunogenic before the age of 2, and does not induce immunological memory. Pneumococcal Conjugate vaccines (PCV) were developed to induce long-lasting protection in infants. Antibody responses to PCV (Prevenar®) in children with SCD are similar to the non-SCD population, and are expected to be protective against serotypes covered by the vaccines. Their use has been associated with a marked decline in morbidity and mortality from IPD. A thirteen-valent conjugate vaccine (Prevenar 13®) has now replaced 7-valent PCV in the routine childhood immunization schedule in North America and most of Europe. It includes 6 additional serotypes that are known to cause severe IPD, and should protect against 80–90 % of serotypes causing IPD in most parts of the world. Current UK guidance is Prevenar 13® at 2, 4 and 13 months with Pneumovax given at 2 years of age. Boosters of Pneumovax are given every 5 years. Although pneumococcal antibody titres can be monitored to confirm response and predict when booster doses are needed, it is not clear how these relate to protection against IPD, and we do not recommend routine testing.

In Sub-Saharan Africa Prevenar 13® or an alternative high valent vaccine could substantially reduce morbidity and mortality in infants and young children with SCD.

It is likely that these vaccines, in combination with regular boosters of Pneumovax in older children, will reduce IPD rates still further, and one wonders whether oral penicillin prophylaxis is still needed for SCD children who are fully vaccinated. However, reports of IPD due to non-vaccine serotypes warrant caution in this respect.

Hemophilus Influenzae Type b and Meningococcal Vaccination

Hemophilus influenzae type b infections include pneumonia and meningits and were responsible for significant morbidity and mortality in children with SCD. These are very rarely encoutered now, since Hib conjugate vaccine was introduced. In developed countries, this is given as part of the childhood vaccination schedule.

Meningococccal group C conjugate vaccine was introduced in 1999 and is also now included in routine childhood immunization schedules. Group B is the most common cause of meningococcal meningitis, and the recent introduction of group B specific vaccines will hopefully result in better protection and control of this serious infection.

Other Vaccinations and Travel Advice

Influenza vaccination: Patients with SCD are at increased risk of serious complications as a consequence of influenza. The H1N1 serotype has been associated with severe disease, increased chest complications and profound anemia. Yearly influenza vaccination is recommended for all patients with SCD.

Hepatitis B vaccination: Patients with SCD are very likely to require blood transfusion at some point and this vaccine should be administered to SCD patients to protect against the small risk of transfusion-transmitted hepatitis B infection. Those receiving regular transfusion should have annual testing of antibody titre to Hepatitis B surface antigen to ensure adequate protection. A booster should be recommended if the titre is inadequate for protection.

Travel advice: Patients with SCD should receive appropriate travel vaccinations as recommended for area of travel, including Meningitis ACWY in high areas.

Bibliography

Booth C, Inusa B, Obaro SK. Infection in sickle cell disease: a review. Int J of Infect Dis. 2010;14:e2–e12.

Davies JM, Lewis MPN, Wimperis J, et al. Review of guidelines for the prevention and treatment of infection in patients with an absent or dysfunctional spleen: prepared on behalf of the British Committee for Standards in Hematology by a Working Party of the Hemato-Oncology Task Force. Br J Haematol. 2011;155:308–17.

Gaston MH, Verter JI, Woods G, et al. Prophylaxis with oral penicillin in children with sickle cell anemia. A randomized trial. N Engl J Med. 1986;314(25):1593–9.

Chapter 13 Gastroenterological Complications

Introduction

Gastroenterological symptoms such as abdominal pain, nausea, vomiting, jaundice, diarrhoea, constipation and weight loss are common, and can be due to complications of SCD or to other common medical conditions, some of which are more frequent in SCD. Table 13.1 lists the most important gastroenterological complications together with their clinical features, laboratory and radiological findings.

Abdominal Crisis (Girdle Syndrome, Mesenteric Sickling)

The abdomen is a common site of pain during acute painful crisis, particularly in children. A more severe form of abdominal crisis is sometimes referred to as 'girdle syndrome', the clinical and radiological features of which are listed in Table 13.1.

Incidence

In our experience girdle syndrome is commoner in children and usually develops during the course of an acute painful crisis.

J. Howard, P. Telfer, *Sickle Cell Disease in Clinical Practice*, In Clinical Practice, DOI 10.1007/978-1-4471-2473-3_13,

Table 13.1 Gastroenterological complications of sickle cell disease-clinical features, laboratory and radiological findings.

	Clinical features	Investigations
Directly related to SCD		
Abdominal sickle crisis ('girdle crisis')	History: Acute onset diffuse abdominal pain and tenderness, often associated with bony pain. Examination: abdominal distension, scanty bowel sounds.	Reduced Hb with reticulocytosis. AXR : Distended small and large bowel loops.
Acute splenic sequestration(See Chap. 11)	History: Acute onset left upper quadrant pain, lethargy . Examination: Pallor, jaundice, spleen palpable and becoming larger, often tender.	Reduced Hb with reticulocytosis.
	Usual presentation is in infants, but also in older children and adults with milder phenotypes of SCD	AUS (not essential if diagnosis obvious): Enlarged spleen
Acute hepatic sequestration	History: Acute onset right upper quadrant pain, fatigue, often associated with an acute painful crisis. Examination: pallor, jaundice, abdominal distension, liver palpable and rapidly enlarging.	Reduced Hb with reticulocytosis. Increased bilirubin, increased AST, ALT, Alk Phos, gamma GT.
	Seen in older children, adolescents and adults	AUS: Enlarged liver

Hepatic crisis/ hepatopathy/ intrahepatic cholestasis	Acute, sub-acute or chronic presentation. Features may be similar or overlapping with acute hepatic sequestration. Commoner in older adults	Reduced Hb with reticulocytosis. Very high bilirubin, and increased AST, ALT, Alk Phos, gamma GT persisting during steady state. AUS: Enlarged liver, intrahepatic ducts may be distended, with thickened irregular walls.
Causes indirectly related to SCD		
Gall-stone related problems: Acute biliary colic, obstructive jaundice, acute cholecystisis, acute pancreatitis	History: Right upper quadrant or epigastric pain, may be colicy. Dark urine, pale stool. Examination: Jaundice. May have fever, pallor. Epigastric and right upper quadrant tenderness	Increased bilirubin, increased AST, ALT, Alk Phos, gamma GT. Amylase raised in acute pancreatitis. AUS: Gallstone (s) in gallbladder and/ or biliary tree. Thickened edematous gallbladder wall, dilated intrahepatic and/ or extrahepatic bile ducts. Pancreas may appear inflamed
Gastritis, peptic ulceration	Predominantly epigastric pain. May be episodic and predominantly at night. May be a history of chronic use of non-steroidal anti-inflammatory drugs	Hematology and biochemistry usually unchanged from steady state. Normal AUS. Gastritis or ulcer demonstrated on upper GI endoscopy

(continued)

Table 13.1 (continued)

	Clinical features	Investigations
Constipation	Common in children and adults and may be the sole cause of abdominal pain. May be related to diet, opioid analgesic use, pica, or abdominal sickling	AXR shows faecal loading, but not advised routinely because of radiation dose
Acute pyelonephritis	Fever, loin pain and tenderness	Perturbation of steady state hematology and biochemistry tests if accompanied by disseminated sepsis or intercurrent acute crisis

AXR abdominal X ray, *AUS* abdominal ultrasound, *AST* aspartate transaminase, *Alk Phos* alkaline phosphatase, *gamma GT* gamma glutamine transaminase, *GI* gastrointestinal

Etiology

It is thought to be due to vaso-occlusion and sequestration in the small vessels of the mesentery, giving rise to abnormal bowel perfusion, transient dysfunction and pain due to ischemia.

Clinical Features

Pain may be restricted to the abdomen, but it is often accompanied by bone pain in the limbs, chest and/or back. There may be additional gastro-intestinal symptoms such as nausea, anorexia and patients usually recognise the pain as being similar to an acute painful crisis. This contrasts with presentations due to a surgical cause, where the pain is recognised as different.

There may be a distended abdomen with very scanty or absent bowel sounds and dilated bowel on abdominal X-ray. The large bowel tends to be the predominant site of dilatation, and this is often accompanied by faecal loading in the distal colon (Figure 13.1). There is usually a drop in hemoglobin with reticulocytosis, presumably reflecting increased hemolysis and mesenteric sequestration of red cells.

Management

Surgical intervention is not required, but surgical colleagues should see the patient in order to familiarize themselves with the complication and to provide advice about conservative measures. Patients should be placed nil by mouth, and a naso-gastric tube inserted. They should have intravenous hydration (but not hyper-hydration), and it is probably sensible to use broad spectrum antibiotics covering gut organisms, even if not clinically septic. They require parenteral analgesia via patient- or nurse-controlled analgesia

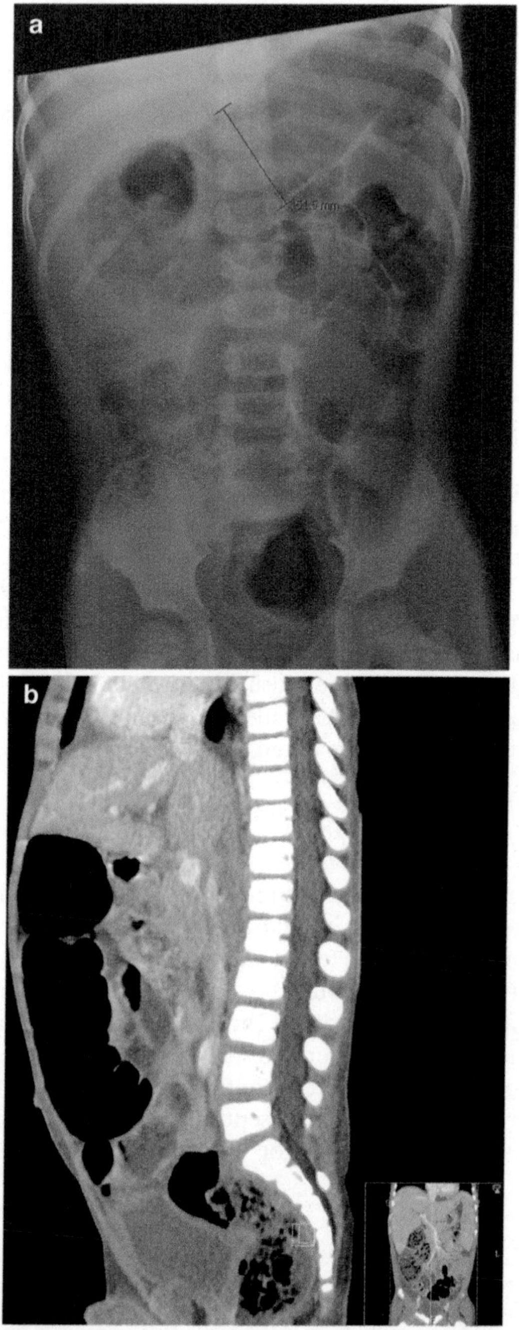

devices. Constipation should be actively managed with suppository or enema. If the hemoglobin level is reduced (<55 g/l) we would recommend initial simple transfusion. This may need to be followed by an urgent exchange transfusion to bring HbS to below 30 % if the condition is severe or complicated by acute chest syndrome.

Colitis

There are case reports of acute ischemic colitis in patients with SCD, thought to be due to bowel infarction secondary to vaso-occlusion.

In addition we have several patients with a diagnosis of ulcerative colitis, who have been managed jointly with specialists in inflammatory bowel disease. Patients typically present with a sudden onset of severe abdominal pain, abdominal distension and bloody stool. Histology of biopsy or colectomy samples in these patients is generally typical of ulcerative colitis without unusual features. Patients should be managed with standard medical therapy. Adequate hydration and analgesia should be ensured. Transfusion or exchange transfusion may be required for acute presentations requiring surgical intervention.

Gallstone-Related Problems

Incidence

Asymptomatic gallbladder disease is very common in older children and adults. Gallstones can be detected by ultrasound examination in about 30 % of adolescents with HbSS, and in over 50 % of adults. The prevalence is lower (around 17 %) in

FIGURE. 13.1 Abdominal X ray (**a**) and CT (**b**) of a 5-year-old child with sickle β^+ thalassemia and girdle syndrome. The large bowel is significantly dilated and there is also fecal loading in the distal colon

HbSC and HbS β thalassemia. Patients with high bilirubin levels in steady state, high hemolytic rate or with Gilbert's syndrome are at increased risk of developing gallstones.

Pathophysiology

Bilirubin is a biochemical product of the breakdown of heme. In hemolytic anemia, breakdown is accelerated and consequently plasma bilirubin levels are often elevated and the patient is jaundiced. Bilirubin is insoluble in water, but it is modified in the liver to a soluble form by conjugation with glucuronide. This can be more easily excreted via the bile and urine. The enzyme hepatic uridine diphosphate-glucuronosyltransferase (UDPGT) is responsible for bilirubin conjugation. Gilbert's Syndrome is a common inherited condition in which UDPGT activity is reduced, and is characterized by episodes of jaundice and high levels of serum unconjugated bilirubin. Patents with Gilbert's Syndrome can be identified by genetic analysis of the gene *UGT1A1* where the defect appears to be a variable expansion of the promoter region.

It has been suggested that gallbladder 'sludge', sometimes detectable on ultrasound examination in younger patients with SCD, is a precursor to gallstone formation, although this remains unproven. Gallstones are usually of the pigmented variety and are black in colour (Figure 13.2). They are composed of bilirubin and calcium carbonate, may be single or multiple and are often packed tightly together, occupying most of the gallbladder volume.

Clinical Features

Asymptomatic gallstones or gallbladder sludge are sometimes diagnosed incidentally when abdominal ultrasound is requested for another reason. More commonly, they are identified during investigation of non-specific abdominal pain.

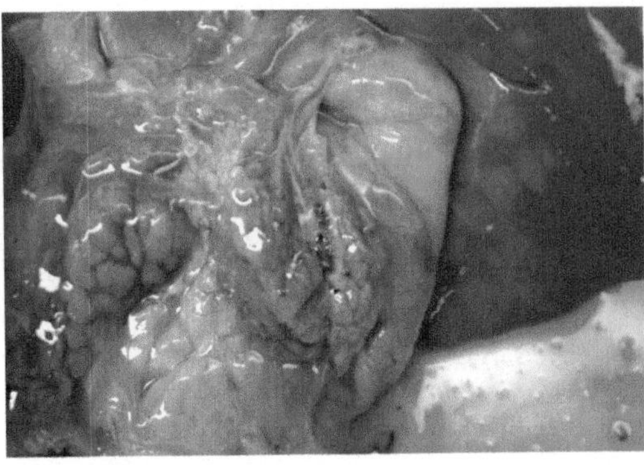

FIGURE 13.2 Pigment gall stones shown in the common bile duct at post mortem. The patient had acute pancreatitis with impaction of a gallstone at the origin of the pancreatic duct

The typical pain of biliary colic is severe, epigastric or right hypochondrial, colicy and often precipitated by food with a high fat-content. Pain usually resolves after an hour or two. Acute cholecystitis (inflammation of the gall bladder) is characterized by more severe, prolonged pain in the same area, combined with nausea, vomiting and jaundice. Patients generally seek urgent medical attention with these symptoms, and on examination, may be darkly jaundiced, with right upper quadrant pain, tenderness and a positive Murphy's sign (heightened tenderness to palpation in the right hypochondrium with inspiration). More rarely, the condition is complicated by high fever, shock and/or features of an acute abdomen. A severe clinical picture like this suggests that there may be an impacted stone in the biliary tree or at the ampulla, associated with cholangitis, cholecystitis or pancreatitis.

Investigations

Liver function tests and abdominal ultrasound (AUS) examination are essential first line investigations (**See** Table 13.1,

Figs. 13.3 and 13.4). In patients with evidence of obstructive jaundice and/or dilated bile ducts on AUS, magnetic resonance cholangio-pancreatography (MRCP) is the best and least invasive means of studying the anatomy of the biliary tree and is helpful for obtaining a more detailed view of the gallbladder and liver (Figure 13.5). Endoscopic or surgical intervention can then be planned on the basis of MRCP findings.

Management

Asymptomatic gall bladder disease does not need intervention. Acute complications related to gallstones should be managed jointly with a hepatobiliary team, which includes specialists in radiology, endoscopic and surgical intervention. Patients require suitable analgesia and opiods are often used. Routine supportive care includes intravenous hydration, insertion of a naso-gastric tube and antibiotic cover for enteric organisms.

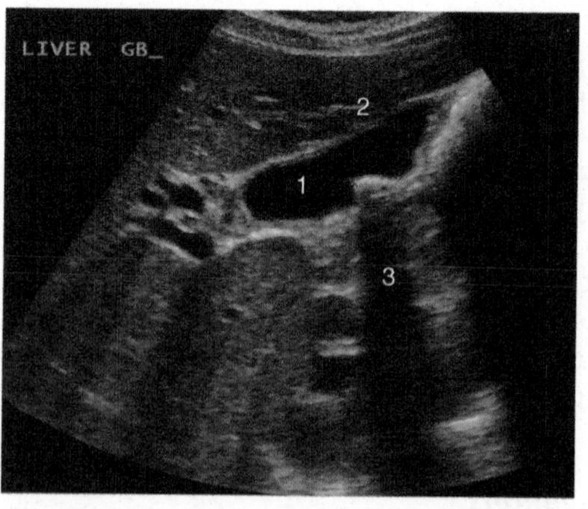

FIGURE 13.3 USS showing a gallstone within the gall bladder. The gallbladder is distended (*1*), the wall of the gallbladder thickened (*2*), and the gallstone is casting an acoustic shadow (*3*)

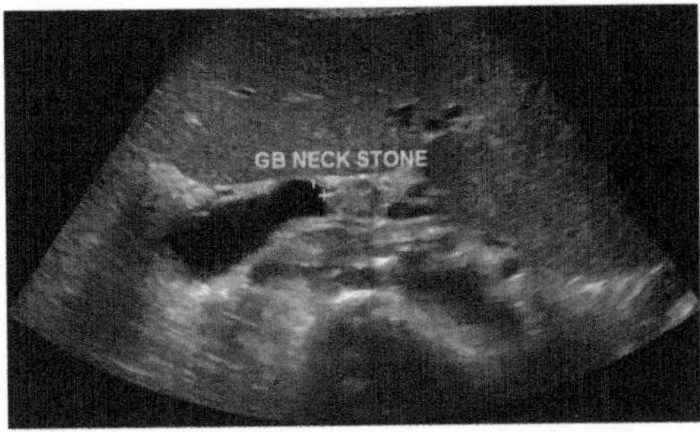

FIGURE 13.4 Ultrasound showing gallstone obstructing the neck of the gallbladder. The patient was male, aged 25 with HbSS, and presented with right upper abdominal pain, vomiting and intense jaundice

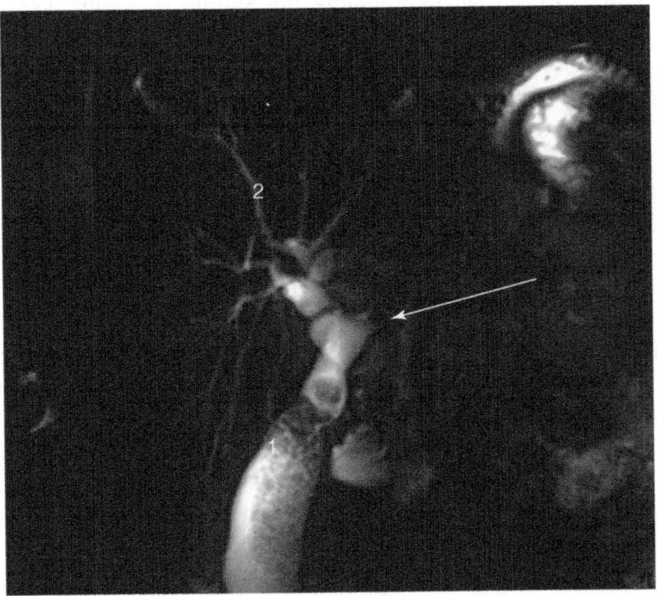

FIGURE 13.5 Magnetic resonance cholangiopancreatography (MRCP) of the same patient, showing dilated gallbladder containing multiple stones (*1*), dilatation of the hepatic ducts (*2*) and a stone obstructing the common bile duct (*arrow*)

Endoscopic retrograde cholangio-pancreatography (ERCP) may be required if there is evidence of bilary obstruction. This has three roles:

1. Visualization of the biliary tree after injection of radio-opaque contrast
2. Creation of a wider orifice at the ampulla to enable passage of impacted stones
3. Physical extraction of stones, often by use of a balloon catheter inserted into the common bile duct.

Acute cholecystitis should be treated with fluids, analgesia and antibiotics. Acute pancreatitis requires intensive medical input with careful monitoring of vital signs, intravenous fluids, oxygen, antibiotics and analgesics with judicious use of intravenous fluids, analgesics and antibiotics. Cholecystectomy is very rarely indicated acutely, but should be planned once the acute episode has resolved. The laparoscopic approach is suitable for most patients. Transfusion or exchange transfusion is not always indicated during an acute episode, but may be necessary because of a drop in hemoglobin level, or as part of the preparative regime for an endoscopic procedure done under sedation or general anaesthetic.

Acute Hepatic Sequestration

This is a well defined acute complication of SCD, in our experience more commonly seen in children and adolescents than in adults. The salient features include acute enlargement of the liver, right upper quadrant pain and tenderness, and an acute drop in hemoglobin level with increased reticulocyte count compared to steady state. These abnormalities are sometimes accompanied by biochemical derangement reflecting hepatic damage and dysfunction. The clinical and laboratory features overlap with 'sickle hepatopathy' (see below). It is not clear whether hepatic sequestration leads to chronic liver disease in later life.

The underlying pathology is assumed to be due to pooling and stasis of sickled erythrocytes within the hepatic sinusoids and venules, and it is sometimes accompanied by an acute painful crisis. There is a rapid drop in hemoglobin level. The condition often resolves rapidly with urgent transfusion, but can progress to acute hepatic failure. Severe episodes require exchange transfusion once hemoglobin level has been restored to steady state with simple transfusion. It is advisable to involve a pediatric or adult hepatologist in the management of these cases.

Sickle Hepatopathy (Intra-Hepatic Cholestasis)

Definition

Neither sickle hepatopathy nor intra-hepatic cholestasis are satisfactory diagnostic terms, but are useful for describing a variety of poorly characterized but increasingly encountered acute and sub-acute hepatic complications seen predominantly in adult patients.

Etiology and Pathophysiology

The underlying pathology is assumed to be pooling and stasis of sickled erythrocytes within the hepatic sinusoids and venules, sometimes combined with additional hepatic pathology due to hemosiderosis, viral hepatitis or autoimmune liver disease. Hypoxic damage leads to areas of parenchymal ischemia, swelling of hepatocytes and occlusion of bile cannaliculi leading to intrahepatic cholestasis. Histological changes are variable, but usually include widespread sickling in the hepatic sinusoids with vascular stasis, areas of hepatic ischemia, severe iron deposition, and sometimes bile duct thickening and proliferation. In later stages there is evidence of fibrosis or cirrhosis.

Clinical Features

Salient features are listed in Table 13.1. The patient can present with mild abdominal pain, hepatomegaly and deranged liver function tests with spontaneous resolution, usually in the context of an acute painful crisis. There may be a more acute presentation with severe right upper quadrant pain together with an enlarging liver, severe jaundice, and often nausea and vomiting. In these cases biochemistry is severely deranged with a mixed cholestatic and hepatitic picture. Severe cases may rapidly progress to acute hepatic decompensation with coagulopathy and ascites.

These clinical features may become a recurrent complication in susceptible patients, with progressive worsening of liver function over time. Often the patient has additional causes of liver damage, including viral hepatitis or autoimmune liver disease. Chronic hepatic iron loading from repeated transfusions is an important cause of chronic liver damage in older patients.

Management

These patients should be managed jointly with a hepatology team. Standard supportive care should be provided. In view of the likely contribution of sickling and vascular stasis within the liver, acute exchange transfusion should be considered. Percutaneous liver biopsy is contraindicated in the acute situation because of a high reported risk of bleeding. Once the acute event has settled, a management plan should be formulated jointly with the hepatology team. In some cases a biopsy (preferably transjugular) is helpful to establish the pathological process, and prioritize management options. Co-morbidities such as transfusional iron overload and chronic hepatitis C infection should be treated. Chronic exchange transfusion is often effective in reducing acute flare-ups and may also reduce the risk of progressive liver damage. There are reports of successful liver transplantation in patients where liver reserve is severely impaired, and with evidence of cirrhosis.

Bibliography

Ahmed S, Shahid RK, Russo LA. Unusual causes of abdominal pain: sickle cell anemia. Best Pract Res Clin Gastroenterol. 2005;19(2):297–310.

Gardner K, Suddle A, Kane P, et al. How we treat sickle hepatopathy and liver transplantation in adults. Blood. 2014;123(15):2302–7.

Chapter 14
Anemia and Sickle Cell Disease

Introduction

Chapter 2 covers normal 'steady state' levels for hemoglobin and their variation with age. The majority of patients with HbSS have steady state hemoglobin levels between 60 and 90 g/l. This anemia is a feature of SCD and is usually well tolerated without the need for routine transfusion. The majority of specialists would not recommend routine treatment for anemia even if the steady state level is <60 g/l but transfusion in these cases may be needed if other chronic complications develop, or if there is an acute drop in hemoglobin during a crisis. Older patients, especially those with pulmonary or cardiac disease, may not tolerate low hemoglobin levels and usually benefit from regular simple transfusion.

Acute Anemia

Clinical Presentation

Increasing anemia may lead to symptoms of tiredness, fatigue and headache. With increasing severity, there is pallor, exercise intolerance, shortness of breath, ankle swelling and eventually circulatory collapse. A slowly progressive anemia is better tolerated than anemia of rapid onset.

J. Howard, P. Telfer, *Sickle Cell Disease in Clinical Practice*, In Clinical Practice, DOI 10.1007/978-1-4471-2473-3_14,

TABLE 14.1 Causes of acute anemia

Cause	Comment
Transient red cell aplasia	Caused by parvovirus B19. Associated with reticulocytopenia
Increased hemolysis	Often accompanies an acute crisis (painful crisis, ACS, girdle syndrome etc.)
Acute splenic sequestration	Splenomegaly, abdominal pain, most common in children
Acute hepatic sequestration	Acute hepatomegaly and abdominal pain
Delayed hemolytic transfusion reaction or hyperhemolysis	Recent history of transfusion (See Chapter 18)
Blood loss	Symptoms of blood loss, iron deficiency
Glucose-6-phosphate dehydrogenase (G6PD) deficiency	Hemolysis following drug administration

Causes and Investigation

The major causes of acute anemia are outlined in Table 14.1, laboratory investigations for determining the cause of anemia in Table 4.3 and a diagnostic algorithm in Fig. 14.1.

Transient Red Cell Aplasia

Pathogenesis

Transient red cell aplasia is caused by parvovirus B19 infection. This is a common infection of childhood usually causing a mild febrile illness and 'slapped cheek syndrome'. The virus selectively targets early erythroid precursors and inhibits erythroblast proliferation and differentiation for 4–8 days (Fig. 14.2). Patients with SCD and other chronic haemolytic

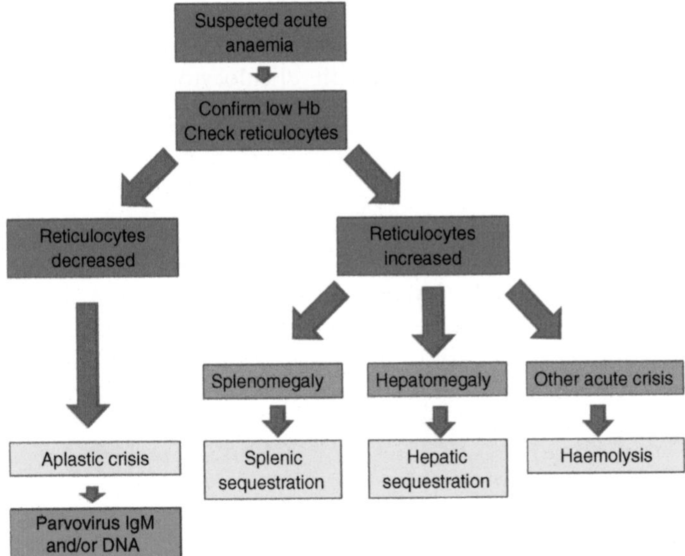

FIGURE 14.1 Algorithm for diagnosis of acute anemia

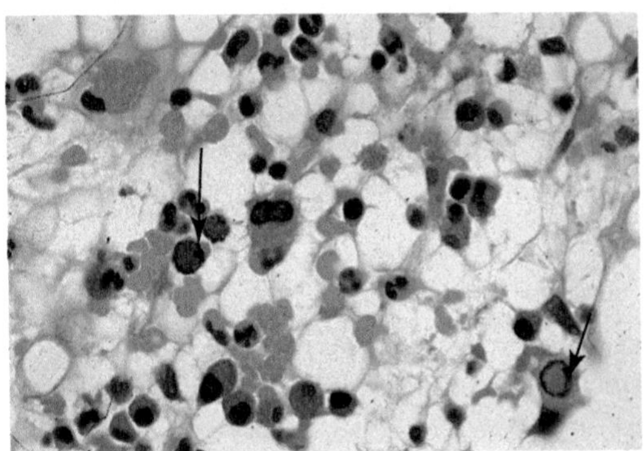

FIGURE 14.2 Parvo B19 infection of red cell precursors (erythroblasts) in the bone marrow, illustrated in a histological section of a bone marrow trephine biopsy. The typical 'lantern' cells (*arrows*) are abnormally enlarged erythroblasts. They have a rim of irregular cytoplasm, and the nucleus contains a perimeter ring of condensed chromatin. Immunohistochemistry (not shown here) can be used to demonstrate intranuclear viral inclusions

conditions require enhanced red cell production to compensate for diminished red cell survival and may consequently develop a profound anemia with reticulocytopenia.

Epidemiology

Presence of anti-parvovirus B19 IgG antibodies in the serum indicates past exposure. Rates of past exposure have been reported at 26 % by 5 years and 73 % by 21 years. A 5-year study in the US reported an incidence rate for transient red cell aplasia secondary to parvovirus B19 of 11.3 events per 100 patient years, and noted that 37.5 % of patients do not develop symptomatic anemia.

Clinical Presentation

Acute parvovirus infection in SCD is frequently associated with a febrile illness and sometimes an acute painful crisis, but it is often asymptomatic. Several family members may be affected. It is usually self limiting and patients will recover within 3–5 days. Occasionally, it is associated with acute splenic sequestration, acute chest syndrome and less commonly stroke or nephrotic syndrome.

Diagnosis

Diagnosis is confirmed by the presence of IgM antibodies to parvovirus B19 (note that IgG antibodies indicate past infection), and/or parvovirus DNA in serum.

Treatment

Patients with a significant fall in Hb (usually >20–30 g/l) require transfusion as soon as possible, aiming to return their Hb to the steady state level. The hemoglobin level and reticulocyte count should be monitored daily to ensure a return to normal values. Occasionally a second transfusion is required. If the patient has had contact with family members or friends with SCD, these contacts should be monitored for viral symptoms and warned about the risks of anemia. During admission to hospital, it is advisable to isolate the patient to minimise the risk of transmission to other patients and pregnant staff. Vaccination against parvovirus B19 would be beneficial as part of the prophylaxis offered to patients with SCD, but unfortunately is not yet available.

Glucose-6-Phosphate Dehydrogenase (G6PD) Deficiency

Deficiency of this enzyme increases erythrocyte susceptibility to oxidant-related damage and haemolysis. Mutations in the gene encoding G6PD are common in Black populations, but generally the deficiency is less severe than in Mediterranean and Asian subjects. It is an X-linked condition, affecting males. Female carriers are less likely to suffer clinical consequences. It is not unusual for G6PD deficiency to be inherited together with SCD, but in most circumstances it does not appear to affect the SCD phenotype significantly, and reports of worse outcomes are inconsistent. In common with any G6PD deficient individual, acute intravascular haemolysis can be precipitated by exposure to agents which provoke oxidant stress. These include certain drugs (including quinolone antibiotics and some anti-malarials), chemicals and fava beans. In our experience, exposure to napthalene in mothballs (used for preservation of clothes) is quite common in SCD families and is a potent oxidant agent. Infection can also sometimes provoke a haemolytic episode.

We recommend that all SCD patients are tested for G6PD deficiency on first booking in the clinic. SCD patients who are G6PD deficient should be issued with a card indicating the diagnosis, and counseled about avoiding agents known to provoke haemolysis (a list of these is available in haematology textbooks and in the British National Formulary). The family doctor should also be informed of the diagnosis.

Chronic Anemia

It is quite common to observe a progressive drop in steady state hemoglobin level during follow-up, with or without increasing symptoms of anemia. Chronic progressive anemia requires full investigation. The cause may be related to a deterioration in SCD, but might also be due to an unrelated condition. Most of these conditions are described elsewhere in the book. In the case of children, causes to consider include progressive hypersplenism, iron and folate deficiency. For adults, in addition to the above, progressive renal impairment is an important cause. Primary haematological disorders may need to be excluded, and occasionally bone marrow examination is required to make a diagnosis.

Bibliography

Smith-Whitely K, et al. Epidemiology of human parvovirus B19 in children with sickle cell disease. Blood. 2004;103(2):422–7.

Chapter 15
Leg Ulceration

Incidence

Leg ulcers are common in SCD. The incidence ranges from 2.5 to 25 % in the US and 30–75 % in Jamaica. They are more common in men and in patients with low steady state hemoglobin and high hemolytic rate. The most frequent sites are the medial and lateral aspects of the ankle, but they can also affect the heel and dorsum of the foot and can be circumferential.

Pathogenesis

Leg ulceration is thought to be related to impaired microvascular circulation and vaso-occlusion in the small dermal vessels. This is most likely to cause problems in the peripheries of the lower limbs, where circulation is more prone to becoming compromised, and where, in SCD, tissue oxygen levels are particularly low. Ulcers may occur spontaneously or secondary to trauma such as from an insect bite, or through wearing inadequate footwear. Other contributory factors are venous incompetence, peripheral edema, abnormal autonomic vascular control and decreased oxygenation. Low nitric oxide levels probably also have a role in provoking vascular dysfunction. Biopsy of involved skin may show microvascular changes

J. Howard, P. Telfer, *Sickle Cell Disease in Clinical Practice*, In Clinical Practice, DOI 10.1007/978-1-4471-2473-3_15,

including intimal proliferation, neovascularization and perivascular proliferation similar to the changes seen in diabetic or vascular ulcers.

Clinical Presentation/Course

The typical established ulcer is round, with raised margins, and a deep base containing necrotic slough, often with surrounding hyperpigmentation. It is not unusual for patients to present after weeks or months of self-management. Leg ulcers in SCD are almost invariably painful and neuropathic pain is common. Stiffness and decreased range of movement in the ankle joint is seen in over 50 % of cases. Complications include superinfection, osteomyelitis, psychosocial disturbance and deterioration in quality of life. Whilst early treatment can be effective, delays may lead to development of large, persistent ulcers. It is not unusual for a large, deep ulcer to require several years to heal, with a high risk of recurrence after minimal trauma.

Diagnosis and Investigation

This is a clinical diagnosis, however complicating conditions should be excluded as these will influence response to treatment. Microbiological swabs should be taken to exclude secondary infection. It may also be appropriate to assess for lower limb venous incompetence, and to exclude underlying osteomyelitis with X-ray or MR scan. Zinc deficiency has been associated with leg ulceration and we recommend checking zinc levels and instituting replacement therapy if required.

Treatment

Most leg ulcer treatment in the UK is now provided in community clinics.

Treatment options can be divided into supportive care, topical treatments, dressings and bandaging, surgical interventions and systemic medications. Initial supportive care includes adequate analgesia and basic ulcer care. Enforced bed rest can help speed the healing process, but is often difficult to sustain. The majority of patients will need opiate analgesia and agents such as gabapentin or pregabalin may be useful for treatment of neuropathic pain. Patients often have abnormal gait and ankle exercises may be helpful.

Topical antibiotics may be needed if there is evidence of infection and parenteral or oral antibiotics are occasionally needed for the treatment of systemic infection or osteomyelitis. Topical opiates have also shown some efficacy. Hyperbaric oxygen and topical growth factors have been used, but need further investigation.

Compression bandaging has an important role in treatment through improving venous return. Compression can be 'long stretch' or 'short stretch', the latter is non elasticated and only squeezes when the patient walks so is more comfortable and easier to apply. There are new bandages available with Velcro strapping which are easily adjusted by the patient, but these are more costly. Compression hosiery can be used acutely and also to prevent recurrence. This can be circular or flat weave, the former gives all over compression, but the latter has decreased elasticity and is better tolerated. Various dressings have been used, some with zinc-oxide impregnation or with anti-infective properties.

Surgical interventions have been used with mixed results, but review by an experienced plastic surgery team can be beneficial. Surgical treatments include debridement, split-thickness skin grafts or pinch grafts and the use of myocutaneous flaps. Our own experience with skin grafting has not been encouraging. We have generally recommended a period of regular transfusion of several months around the procedure, with the aim of increasing local tissue perfusion.

Systemic therapies include zinc replacement, which should be given to patients with zinc deficiency. A trial of blood transfusion therapy is helpful in some patients, and is likely to improve tissue perfusion and contribute to improved healing. Other treatments which have been tried include topical sodium nitrate, hyperbaric oxygen, arginine, L-carnitine and erythropoietin but these need further investigation. The role of hydroxyurea is not clear. It is associated with leg ulceration in patients with myeloproliferative disorders, and although this is not a consisitent finding in long term studies of hydroxyurea in SCD, some patients do seem to suffer more problems with ulceration. For patients who experience a recurrence or worsening of existing ulceration whilst on hydroxyurea it may be worth reducing the dose or interrupting therapy.

Prevention of ulcers is an important part of general health care, especially for patients with recurrent disease. Patients should be careful to avoid minor trauma to the legs (including cannulation of veins around the ankle) and use emollients to prevent cracking of the skin. Support stockings may be appropriate for those with a history of recurrent ulceration.

Bibliography

Cumming V, King L, Fraser R, Serjeant G, Reid M. Venous incompetence, poverty and lactate dehydrogenase in Jamaica are important predictors of leg ulceration in sickle cell disease. B J Haematol. 2007;142:119–25.

Halabi-Tawil M, Lionnet F, Girot R, Bachmeyer C, Levy PP, Aractingi S. Sickle cell leg ulcers: a frequently disabling complication and a marker of severity. B J Dermatol. 2008;158:339–44.

Minniti CP, Eckman J, Sebastiani P, Steinberg MH, Ballas SK. Leg ulcers in sickle cell disease. Am J Hematol. 2010;85(10):831–3.

Trent JT, Kirsner RS. Leg ulcers in sickle cell disease. Adv Skin Wound Care. 2004;17(8):410–6.

Part III
Practical Issues in the Management of Sickle Cell Disease

Chapter 16
Management of Pregnancy

Introduction

In the 21st century, women with sickle cell disease (SCD) should expect to have successful pregnancies and healthy babies. This requires management by a multidisciplinary team which has shared knowledge, experience and expertise in managing high-risk pregnancies. The team usually includes the obstetrician, obstetric anesthetist, midwife, hematologist and sickle cell nurse specialist. If this resource is not available in a local hospital, we recommend that the pregnancy is jointly managed with a regional specialist center.

The reported rates of maternal and fetal complications vary considerably between studies, but there is no doubt that they are significantly higher than in a normal pregnancy (Table 16.1). This applies to all genotypes of SCD, although women with HbSS are most at risk. Earlier series emphasized a very high rate of maternal mortality, but this is not the case nowadays, especially in large specialized centers. The frequency and severity of acute painful crises requiring hospitalization is high, particularly in the later stages of pregnancy, and this also applies to women with a mild phenotype.

Figure 16.1 illustrates the expected abnormality on the maternal side of the circulation and the normal appearance on the fetal side of the placental circulation.

J. Howard, P. Telfer, *Sickle Cell Disease in Clinical Practice*, In Clinical Practice, DOI 10.1007/978-1-4471-2473-3_16,

TABLE 16.1 Maternal and fetal complications

Maternal complications	Fetal complications
Acute painful crisis and acute chest syndrome	Miscarriage (throughout pregnancy)
Infection (especially UTI)	Premature labour
Thromboembolism	Perinatal morbidity and mortality
Pre-eclampsia and pregnancy induced hypertension	Stillbirth
Increased rate of Cesarean section	Fetal growth restriction
Hospitalization during pregnancy	
Maternal mortality	

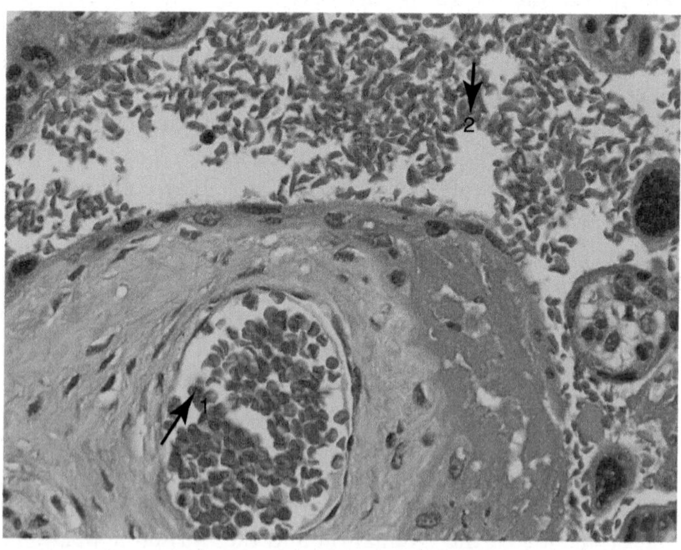

FIGURE 16.1 Placental histology in HbSS. The fetal blood vessel contains normal red cells (1) and the maternal blood vessel contains sickled red cells (2)

Preconceptual Care

Although pregnancies are sometimes unplanned, prior discussion and planning enables optimization of maternal health, and enables a pre-conceptual risk assessment. Knowledge of the father's hemoglobinopathy status is obviously essential for counselling about the risk of SCD for the baby. If mother has pre-existing red cell alloantibodies arising from transfusion or previous pregnancies, there may be a risk of hemolytic disease of the newborn (HDN). Some medications (for instance hydroxyurea, iron chelating agents) are contraindicated in pregnancy as they may cause damage to the developing fetus.

Discussions concerning reproductive options, pregnancy risks and the impact of SCD on mother and baby should be part of the annual review for women of childbearing age. Women who are planning pregnancy should have a fresh evaluation for the chronic complications of SCD which may adversely affect their health during pregnancy. These include pulmonary hypertension, chronic lung disease, renal disease and retinopathy. For women with significant iron overload, a period of intensive iron chelation therapy is essential in order to bring body iron stores down to safe levels prior to conception.

Medications and vaccination history should also be reviewed and potentially embryotoxic drugs stopped. In the case of hydroxyurea, this may entail a discussion of alternative means of controlling acute sickle cell crises during pregnancy. Although there is no clear evidence of benefit of antibiotic prophylaxis in pregnant women with SCD, we recommend oral penicillin V is continued. Folic acid is beneficial in the prevention of neural tube defects and as women with SCD have increased folate requirements they should continue folic acid 5 mg daily prior to and during pregnancy.

The father's hemoglobinopathy status should be confirmed by viewing a laboratory report rather than relying on a verbal report. At-risk couples should receive counselling and advice about reproductive options including preimplantation genetic diagnosis and prenatal diagnosis.

Antenatal Care

Women with SCD should be advised to inform their hematologist as soon as they become pregnant. It is not unknown for a woman to conceive whilst taking hydroxyurea. Whilst these pregnancies have generally resulted in normal babies, there is evidence of teratogenicity in animal models. On current evidence the risk is not sufficient to advise termination but the woman should be offered a detailed anomaly scan at 20 weeks.

There is evidence that low dose aspirin (75 mg) can decrease the risk of pre-eclampsia in high risk pregnancies and although there is no specific evidence in SCD, the authors recommend low dose aspirin in women with no contra-indications to its use.

Pregnant women with SCD should be referred to a multidisciplinary high-risk pregnancy team. Many large centres have set up joint haematology-obstetric clinics and these are ideal for co-ordinated management. We recommend monthly review to 24 weeks, fortnightly to 34 weeks and weekly thereafter. Regular monitoring includes blood pressure and urinalysis. Ultrasound monitoring should be carried out routinely in early pregnancy, and 4 weekly from 24 weeks to monitor fetal growth and amniotic fluid volume. If there is evidence of fetal growth restriction obstetricians may need to consider early delivery. Uterine artery Doppler scanning is also useful for assessing placental blood flow and can be included in the assessment schedule.

Acute pain crises are common during pregnancy, occurring in up to 50 % of women. Mild sickle pain can be managed in the community with rest, fluids and simple analgesics, but pregnant women who present with acute severe pain should be admitted. Obstetric units should have clear protocols for the emergency care of women with SCD including regular monitoring of maternal and fetal vital signs. Intravenous hydration, anti-emetics and laxatives are needed more frequently than outside of pregnancy. The analgesia protocol can be similar to what is used in the non-pregnant patient, however, non-steroidal anti-inflammatory drugs should be avoided because of the risk of premature closure of the fetal ductus arteriosus. It is also advisable to avoid using opioids for which there is limited experience of use in pregnancy, such as oxycodone and fentanyl.

Transfusion During Pregnancy

Blood requirements are broadly the same as outside of pregnancy, however, the UK National Blood Service currently recommends that blood for pregnant women should be negative for CMV.

Although transfusion reduces the incidence of painful crises it does not impact on the incidence of other maternal and fetal complications, and we do not recommend transfusion for all pregnant women throughout pregnancy. Those who are already on a transfusion programme should continue, and transfusion can also be considered for women with an increased frequency of acute painful crises, for those who have been maintained on hydroxyurea prior to pregnancy, and women with severe anemia in steady state (Hb <70 g/L).

In the acute setting, simple transfusion should be used for managing acute anemia and exchange transfusion for the treatment of acute chest syndrome or stroke. Exchange transfusion can be performed as a manual or automated procedure although there is a preference for automated exchange as it is easier to ensure isovolemia.

Intrapartum Care

If there are no obstetric contraindications and the fetus is developing normally, we recommend that the pregnancy should be allowed to progress to term, anticipating a spontaneous labour and normal vaginal delivery. Whilst there is no randomized data on the optimal time for delivery, the high rate of late pregnancy complications have led many groups to encourage delivery by 38–40 weeks. Induction of labour should be considered after 38 + 6 weeks and certainly at 39 + 6 weeks, or earlier if there is evidence of poor fetal growth. The need for Cesarean section should be based on standard guidelines.

Women should be kept warm and given adequate fluids and inhaled oxygen as needed. Continuous fetal monitoring is mandatory. Analgesia during labour should be tailored to the individual, taking into account the usual analgesia plan for managing acute sickle crisis pain, and the degree of opiod tolerance from past exposure. Pethidine should be avoided because of the risk of fits. Regional analgesia is preferred for caesarean section because of the increased risks associated with general anaesthesia in SCD. Routine blood transfusion is not recommended prior to caesarean section, but should be considered when hemoglobin level has dropped to below 70 g/l or more than 20 g/l below the patient's baseline. If the patient is known to have red cell alloantibodies, blood should be cross-matched early, in anticipation of the requirement.

Postpartum Care

Adequate hydration, oxygenation and analgesia should be maintained post-partum. We recommend daily medical assessment by the hematology team, including a thorough examination of the chest to evaluate the risk of acute chest crisis, which is high in the post-partum period. Patients on hydroxyurea prior to pregnancy can restart once breastfeeding is finished. Provision of ongoing blood transfusion for several months after delivery can be considered for patients who have required transfusion during pregnancy particularly if they have had recurrent painful crises.

Thromboprophylaxis

Although the risk of venous thromboembolism is probably increased slightly in pregnant women with SCD, this is not a sufficient reason to give antenatal prophylaxis if there are no additional risk factors. We recommend that women are assessed antenatally for thrombotic risk using national guidelines, such as those produced by the Royal College of Obstetricians and Gynaecologists (RCOG). Additional risk factors include a previous or family history of venous thromboembolism, inherited thrombophilia, other medical co-morbidities, age over 35 years, raised body mass index (BMI), smoking and pre-eclampsia. We recommend that women are given prophylactic dose low molecular weight heparin if they are admitted to hospital during pregnancy. Antiembolic stockings are recommended during labour. The requirement for post natal thromboprophylaxis should be assessed using standard guidelines. In the absence of additional risk factors low molecular weight heparin should be given for 7 days after a vaginal delivery and 6 weeks after an emergency caesarean section.

Bibliography

Sickle Cell Disease in Pregnancy, Management of (Green-top 61). Royal College of Obstetricians and Gynaecologists. 2011. www.rcog.org.uk/womens-health/clinical-guidance.

Thrombosis and Embolism during Pregnancy and the Puerperium, Reducing the Risk (Green-top 37a). Royal College of Obstetricians and Gynaecologists. 2009. www.rcog.org.uk/womens-health/clinical-guidance.

Chapter 17
Surgical Management

Introduction

Surgery is often necessary in patients with SCD, the most common procedures being tonsillectomy and splenectomy in children and laparoscopic cholecystecomy and joint replacement surgery in adults. There is an increased risk of surgical complications (infection, thrombosis), and complications related to SCD (painful sickle crisis and acute chest syndrome). For optimal outcomes, it is important to co-ordinate care given by surgeons, anesthetists and hematologists. The medical condition of the patient should be optimized before surgery, and planned procedures should be postponed if the patient is febrile or has a sickle cell crisis.

Preoperative Screening for SCD and Carrier Status

Whilst most patients will be aware that they have SCD, it is prudent to ensure testing has been done on all non-Northern Europeans prior to surgery. For routine surgery this can be done in the preoperative assessment clinic, by requesting full blood count, film and haemoglobinopathy screen (by HPLC or alternative laboratory method). Patients who are

J. Howard, P. Telfer, *Sickle Cell Disease in Clinical Practice*,
In Clinical Practice, DOI 10.1007/978-1-4471-2473-3_17,

identified to have SCD should be discussed with the hematology and anesthetic team and a management plan developed as outlined below. In the emergency setting, where the sickle cell status is not known at the time of surgery, an urgent sickle solubility test, full blood count and haemoglobinopathy screen should be requested, but often the result of the haemoglobinopathy screen will be not be available immediately. A negative sickle solubility test will exclude a sickling disorder. If positive it will not discriminate between carrier or disease status. In this situation the full blood count result and blood film should be reviewed. If the patient has a normal hemoglobin concentration and no history of painful crises then HbSS is unlikely. A normal hemoglobin may be seen in HbSC but the blood film will show characteristic changes. The hematology team should be contacted for advice. If surgery is urgent it should proceed and the patient should be treated as if they have SCD until confirmatory tests are available.

Preoperative Management

All patients with SCD who need general anesthesia should be discussed with their hematologist prior to planned surgery to co-ordinate management. Suggested preoperative investigations are outlined in Table 17.1.

Preoperative review should include assessment of previous analgesia requirements so that recommendations can be made about postoperative pain relief. This is especially important for patients on long term opiates to avoid inadequate postoperative pain management. The review should also include an assessment of end-organ damage (renal disease, pulmonary hypertension, chronic lung disease) as these complications may necessitate more complex perioperative management. For example a patient with chronic lung disease and low baseline oxygen levels may need postoperative admission to a High Dependency Unit for intensive monitoring and/ or postoperative respiratory support.

TABLE 17.1 Preoperative blood tests

Investigation	Purpose
Full blood count	To compare Hb with previous results. Current Hb level is required for decision on pre-operative transfusion
Haemoglobin analysis by HPLC	Recommended for evaluating current pre-transfusion HbS%
Renal function	To assess for sickle nephropathy
Group and antibody screen	To confirm there are no red cell antibodies
Extended red cell phenotype	If this has not previously been done

Preoperative Blood Transfusion

There has been controversy about the role of preoperative blood transfusion in patients with SCD. Whilst early observational studies showed decreased surgical complications if preoperative transfusion was given, other studies were contradictory and also showed increased rates of transfusion related complications in patients receiving pre-operative transfusion. One randomized controlled trial showed no difference in perioperative and postoperative complication rates when aggressive (exchange) transfusion and simple (top-up) transfusion regimes were used, implying that simple (top-up) transfusion was as effective as exchange transfusion in preventing complications. A recent randomized trial (TAPS trial) compared complication rates in patients receiving preoperative simple transfusion (unless Hb was >90 g/l when partial exchange transfusion was used) with no preoperative transfusion in patients with moderate and low risk surgery. This trial showed a clear benefit of preoperative transfusion with a highly significant increase in all complications and in serious adverse events in the non-transfused group. The majority of the serious adverse events were acute chest syndrome, and most of these patients required perioperative or postoperative blood transfusion. Although the trial only included patients with HbSS and HbS β^0 thalassemia and numbers were relatively small, the authors make the following recommendations.

HbSS and HbS β^0 thalassemia:

- Offer all patients preoperative transfusion 2–10 days prior to surgery.
- High risk surgery (neurosurgery, cardiac surgery, complex orthopedic surgery including total hip replacement).
  - Offer an exchange transfusion 2–10 days prior to surgery aiming for a preoperative Hb of 100 g/l and HbS% of <30 %.
- Low or moderate risk surgery (tonsillectomy, splenectomy, cholecystectomy, arthroscopy).
  - If Hb <90 g/l offer a top up transfusion aiming for a preoperative Hb of 100 g/l.
  - If Hb is >90 g/l offer a partial exchange transfusion aiming for preoperative Hb of 100 g/l and HbS% of <60 %.
- If patients are already on a regular exchange transfusion programme they should have an exchange timed in the 2–10 days prior to surgery.
- In patients with a very severe phenotype and Hb <90 g/l, a preoperative exchange transfusion should be considered.

HbSC and other genotypes:

- In view of the lack of evidence for transfusion in this group the decision for transfusion should be made on a case-by-case basis and guided by the type of surgery to be undertaken and disease severity.
- High-risk surgery (neurosurgery, cardiac surgery, complex orthopedic surgery including total hip replacement).
  - Offer an exchange transfusion 2–10 days prior to surgery aiming for a preoperative Hb of 100 g/l and HbS + C of <30 %.
- Low or moderate risk surgery (tonsillectomy, splenectomy, arthroscopy, laparoscopic surgery).

- If Hb <90 g/l offer a top up transfusion aiming for a preoperative Hb of 100 g/l.
- If Hb is >90 g/l no transfusion unless very severe disease phenotype.

If blood transfusion is not possible (e.g., multiple red cell antibodies or previous hyperhemolysis), erythropoietin and intravenous iron may increase the hemoglobin preoperatively. We have also used hydroxyurea (during a period of 6–8 weeks prior to surgery) in this situation.

Perioperative and Postoperative Care:

- Careful management of fluid balance is essential. Intravenous fluid should be started preoperatively and continued until the patient is drinking freely.
- In view of the high risk of postoperative acute chest syndrome, oxygen saturations on air should be monitored regularly in the postoperative period. The patient should have a careful medical review if the saturations fall below 94 % (or >3 % below baseline). Incentive spirometry (ten deep breaths every 2 hours) should be instituted as soon as practical.
- The patient should be reviewed daily by the surgical and hematology team. Assessment should include the surgical site, complications such as infection, thrombosis and acute sickle crisis. Pain score, opiate side effects and analgesia dosing should be monitored frequently.
- Routine surgical thromboprophylaxis should be prescribed. If there are additional risk factors, thrombo prophylaxis should be intensified.

Emergency Surgery

In the emergency situation the liaison between the surgeon, hematologist and anaesthetist needs to be co-ordinated rapidly and the means of communication with on-call teams should be planned in advance as part of the service protocol. The hematology team should confirm the patient's sickle status, clarify the history of transfusion complications and red cell antibodies and review the history of previous complications of SCD. This will aid decision making about the need for blood transfusion.

For patients with a low steady state Hb level (<80 g/l) a simple transfusion can be given before or during surgery. For a patient with high Hb level (>90 g/l), a preoperative emergency exchange transfusion may be needed. More commonly the emergency surgery will go ahead, with close postoperative monitoring and early postoperative transfusion undertaken if required. If surgery is needed immediately as a life-saving procedure it should be performed and blood transfusion (simple or exchange) can be given intraoperatively or postoperatively.

Regional Anaesthesia

Sickle complications are less likely with spinal or epidural anaesthesia than with general anaesthesia and preoperative transfusion is not usually required unless the phenotype is particularly severe or the patient very anemic (Hb <70 g/l).

Bibliography

Howard J, Malfroy M, Llewelyn C, et al. The Transfusion Alternatives Preoperatively in Sickle Cell Disease (TAPS) study: a randomized controlled multicenter clinical trial. Lancet. 2013;381(9870):930–8.

Vichinsky EP, Haberkern CM, Neumayr L, et al. A comparison of conservative and aggressive transfusion regimens in the perioperative management of sickle cell disease. The Preoperative Transfusion in Sickle Cell Disease Study Group. N Engl J Med. 1995;333(4):206–13.

Chapter 18
Treatment of Sickle Cell Disease

Hydroxyurea

Hydroxyurea (or hydroxycarbamide), is currently the only licensed drug for long-term control of SCD.

Mechanism of Action

Hydroxyurea is a cytostatic agent which depletes the intracellular pool of deoxyribonucleotides required for synthesis and repair of DNA. This action is due to inhibition of the enzyme ribonucleotide reductase. The hematological effects include increases in fetal hemoglobin (HbF), mean cell volume (MCV), and steady state hemoglobin level. These are generally accompanied by a reduction in reticulocytes, white cells and platelets, and in markers of hemolysis including bilirubin and LDH. The reduction in intracellular sickling and in circulating dense red cells can be directly observed by comparing morphology of erythrocytes on the blood film before and during therapy (Fig. 18.1).

Augmentation of fetal hemoglobin is probably the principle mechanism of action, and this is thought to be caused by disruption of erythropoiesis with restriction of cell division in the marrow (stress erythropoiesis). Bone marrow suppression also results in a reduction in leukocyte count, which may

J. Howard, P. Telfer, *Sickle Cell Disease in Clinical Practice*, In Clinical Practice, DOI 10.1007/978-1-4471-2473-3_18,

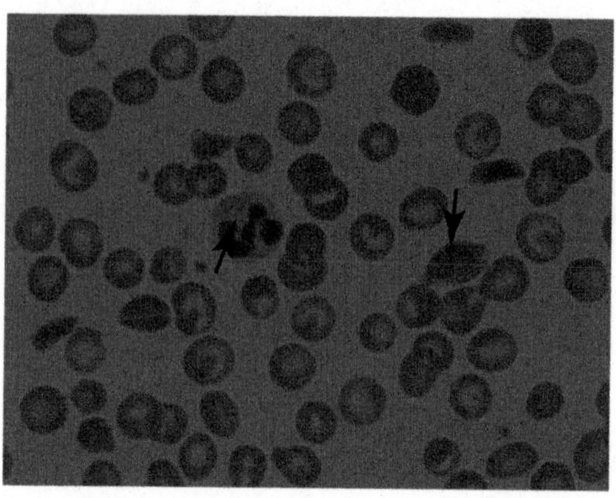

FIGURE 18.1 Blood film of patient with HbSS on hydroxyurea. Sickled cells are seen together with a red cell containing a Howell-Jolly body (*down arrow*). The changes associated with hydroxyurea therapy include macrocytosis (red cells are enlarged, in some cases almost to the size of the neutrophil), and neutrophil hypersegmentation (*up arrow*)

be important since leukocytes are thought to play an important role in initiation of vaso-occlusion (See Chap. 1). The reduction in reticulocyte count and of sickled cells may also contribute to decreased red cell-endothelial interactions important in vaso-occlusion. Hydroxyurea also functions as a nitric oxide donor.

Efficacy

Prevention of Acute Complications

The Multicenter Study of Hydroxyurea (MSH) compared hydroxyurea with placebo in adults with HbSS and more than three acute painful crises per year (not necessarily requiring treatment in hospital). Hydroxyurea was commenced at 15 mg/kg and the dose escalated by 5 mg/kg/day at 12 weekly intervals aiming for maximum tolerated dose (MTD, see below). The trial was halted early, after a significant decrease in acute painful crises was confirmed. The final analysis showed a reduction in annual rate of acute painful crisis by about 50 %. There were also significant reductions in rates of acute chest syndrome and of crises requiring blood transfusion. These clinical effects were mirrored by an increase in HbF and MCV, which became apparent after 8 weeks of therapy and reached a peak at about 40 weeks.

Similar beneficial effects in acute crisis prevention have been shown in pediatric populations. Most recently the BABY-HUG study randomized children at 9–18 months of age to either hydroxyurea or placebo, irrespective of disease severity. The starting dose was 20 mg/kg/day and there was no dose escalation. This trial showed a significant decrease in pain episodes, dactylitis, acute chest syndrome, hospitalization and events requiring transfusion.

Prevention of Chronic Organ Damage

The BABY-HUG study was designed to test the concept that treatment started in infants would prevent or reduce chronic organ damage. The primary outcomes were measures of splenic and renal function (glomerular filtration rate) by radionucleotide scanning. There was no significant effect of hydroxyurea treatment on these measures. The SWiTCH trial examined the role of hydroxyurea in secondary prevention of stroke compared to transfusion. This trial is described in Chap. 7. The authors of the trial concluded that transfusion and chelation remain a better way of managing children with SCD, stroke, and iron overload. The TWiTCH trial is currently examining the role of hydroxyurea compared to transfusion in prevention of first stroke in children with abnormal Transcranial Doppler velocities, and results are awaited eagerly.

These unconvincing results in randomized controlled trials may relate to trial design and to short duration of follow-up. Improvements in organ function have been observed in prospective non-randomized studies. Examples include preservation of splenic function, secondary stroke prevention, lowering of Transcranial Doppler velocities, prevention of silent cerebral infarction, and treatment of pulmonary hypertension. For some of these, there are also studies that have failed to show a benefit of hydroxyurea. Some complications of SCD do not appear to be significantly improved whilst on hydroxyurea therapy, and may even deteriorate. We have noted this with avascular necrosis in childhood, priapism and lower limb ulceration.

The long-term effects of hydroxyurea on chronic organ damage are still not clarified and further randomized controlled studies will be important for refining the indications for therapy in both children and adults. These will be supplemented by long-term observational studies, such as The Long-Term Effects of Hydroxyurea Therapy in Children with Sickle Cell Disease (HUSTLE) which is a single center US study, gathering prospective data on end-organ damage and toxicity in children and planned to continue over at least 20 years.

Improved Life Expectancy

It is reasonable to expect that patients who have a good clinical and hematological response, and who can adhere to therapy in the long-term, will have improved life expectancy. This assumes that there are no unexpected adverse effects which are yet to emerge on long-term follow-up. The improvement could be related both to a reduction in life threatening acute crises, and a reduced risk of progressive organ damage.

So far, three non-randomized, long-term prospective studies provide some evidence supporting a reduction in mortality:

1. Long-term follow-up of patients previously randomized in the MSH study has suggested an improvement in survival associated with the duration of hydroxyurea exposure.
2. Retrospective data from a Brazilian pediatric cohort has shown improved survival in children treated with

hydroxyurea for a median of 2 years with fewer deaths from acute chest syndrome and infections in the treated group.

3. A prospective study from the Laikon Hospital in Athens, Greece in which severely affected adult patients (the majority with HbS β^0 thalassemia) were treated with hydroxyurea and compared with less severely affected patients who were treated in the same center. There was improved survival at 10 years in patients on hydroxyurea compared to standard treatment (86 % compared to 64 %), as well as a decrease in acute painful crisis, acute chest syndrome and hospital admissions in the treated group.

On the other hand, there are studies in which hydroxyurea therapy does not appear to be a significant predictor of survival. Nevertheless, the evidence on reduced mortality may justify use of hydroxyurea in asymptomatic children and adults and for other indications where direct evidence for benefit does not yet exist (for example in patients with a tricuspid jet velocity >2.5 m/s on echocardiography). In order to be clearer on this important issue, more longitudinal follow-up and safety data is urgently required.

Adverse Effects

Although there were initial safety concerns, particularly in the pediatric population, long-term data has so far been reassuring. The HUG-KIDS study, an observational study of 5–16 year olds showed no adverse effects on growth and development. HUSOFT and its extension study, a prospective open-label trial in 6–28 month olds, unselected for disease severity showed very few toxicities. Long-term safety data in adults include the MSH follow-up report, and the Laikon Hospital data. There were no unexpected adverse events reported over 17 years of treatment in these studies. There are important on-going trials, including the HUSTLE study which will report on long-term toxicities in children. These need to be supplemented by prospective national or regional registry data, and we hope that the National Hemoglobinopathy

Register will become a useful instrument for reporting on treatment, efficacy and adverse effects in the UK.

Myelosuppression

Myelosuppression is the most important short-term side effect and requires monitoring with regular blood tests. Although more common with higher doses, the incidence of myelosuppression is variable and can occur in patients who have been on hydroxyurea for many years, indeed there is some evidence that older patients may be more prone to developing myelosuppression at lower doses of hydroxyurea. This may be due to progressive infarction of active marrow and reduced bone marrow reserve in older patients. Trials which have used dose escalation to MTD have shown higher rates of myelosuppression than trials using a 'minimal effective dose' to achieve the therapeutic goal of control of acute painful crisis episodes.

Other Adverse Effects

Other short- to medium term adverse effects include nausea, which usually settles within a few weeks, hyperpigmentation of nails and hair thinning. These are sometimes unacceptable for young people.

Teratogenicity

In vitro hydroxyurea is mutagenic, and hydroxyurea treatment in laboratory animals can cause fetal abnormalities. In clinical experience, the majority of pregnancies where women have been exposed to hydroxyurea have resulted in normal babies. Women and men must be advised to use contraception whilst on hydroxyurea and to stop hydroxyurea at least 3 months before conceiving. If a woman becomes pregnant whilst on hydroxyurea, the drug should be stopped immediately and recommenced only after finishing breastfeeding. Hydroxyurea appears in breast milk at a concentration proportional to the oral dose, and is best avoided during breast feeding.

Effects on Spermatogensis

Sperm motility and sperm count are often decreased during hydroxyurea therapy and do not always return to normal, even several months after cessation. There are reports of long term azospermia in which hydroxyurea has been implicated, but in some cases these are more likely to be due to SCD. Testicular ischaemia and infarction has been suggested as a possible cause of reduced sperm count in men with SCD who have never been treated with hydroxyurea. An expert panel from the National Toxicology Program in the US has expressed concerns about the adverse effects of hydroxyurea on spermatogenesis based on data from young laboratory animals.

In summary, the long-term effects of hydroxyurea on spermatogenesis and male fertility are not yet clear, particularly in the case of boys who start medication at a young age. For post-pubertal males we recommend sperm count and if viable sperm are present, sperm cryopreservation before commencing hydroxyurea treatment. For parents of young children, this uncertainty needs to be communicated as part of the discussion of benefits and risks.

Risk of Malignancy

A potential increased risk of cancer with long-term hydroxyurea therapy has been one of the major reasons for reluctance of clinicians and patients to use hydroxyurea. The theoretical risk relates to its mechanism of action, in particular inhibition of the DNA repair process. There is some evidence from experience with myeloproliferative conditions (which are premalignant disorders of the blood seen mostly in adults) suggesting an increased risk of transformation to acute leukemia associated with hydroxyurea therapy, but this is largely explained by the preferential selection for treatment of more severe cases, which would be more likely to transform anyway.

At least two studies have examined for DNA changes in children taking hydroxyurea, including an ancillary of the BABYHUG study, which looked for chromatid breakages and aberrant recombination events in the immunoglobulin genes, and did not find any convincing *in vitro* evidence of genotoxicity.

In clinical practice, although there are case reports of malignant disease (particularly leukemias) in patients on hydroxyurea, the incidence does not appear to be at a higher frequency than in the general population. With up to 20 years of clinical experience since the first publication of the MSH study, and many thousands of patients from all over the world treated with hydroxyurea, the lack of reports indicating an increased risk of malignancy is reassuring.

Use in Clinical Practice

Indications

Table 18.1 lists suggested indications for hydroxyurea in children and adults.

These indications are discussed in more detail elsewhere under the specific complications. The majority of trials in SCD have been limited to patients with HbSS or included small numbers of patients with other genotypes. A pragmatic approach for HbS β thalassemia and HbSC is to use the same indications as in patients with HbSS.

Patients and families need to be informed about hydroxyurea and its potential benefits, and the information repeated by clinic doctors and nurse specialists as opportunities present themselves, including at the annual review visit. We advise that a clinic-specific patient information sheet is made available to help in reaching a decision on therapy.

Dosing and Monitoring

The starting dose is usually 15 mg/kg. Maximum tolerated dose (MTD) will result in optimal HbF response, and better control of sickling, but at the expense of increased risk of side

TABLE 18.1 Suggested indications for hydroxyurea

Indication	Comments
HbSS	
>2 admissions to hospital per year with acute painful crisis	High-grade evidence, hydroxyurea should be recommended
One or more episodes of acute chest syndrome	High-grade evidence, hydroxyurea should be recommended
Recurrent painful episodes managed at home, but impacting on activity and quality of life	Moderate level evidence, hydroxyurea should be recommended
Severe anemia and high hemolytic rate	Hydroxyurea likely to be of benefit and should considered
HbSS with renal dysfunction or albuminuria	Moderate level evidence. Hydroxyurea should be considered in conjunction with ACEi or ARBs
Chronic lung disease, pulmonary hypertension	Moderate level evidence Hydroxyurea should be considered in conjunction with specific treatment
Recurrent priapism, leg ulceration, retinopathy, raised TR jet velocity	Low level evidence. Trial of hydroxyurea can be considered if risks outweigh the benefits
Secondary stroke prophylaxis	Recommend hydroxyurea if patient is unable to receive blood transfusion
Raised TCD velocity	Recommend hydroxyurea if patient is unable to receive blood transfusion
Generally asymptomatic	Discuss the benefits and risks of hydroxyurea with patient to allow them to reach an informed decision
HbSC and other genotypes	
Features of severe disease (recurrent pain, acute chest syndrome)	Moderate level evidence. Hydroxyurea should be recommended
Asymptomatic or mild disease	Inadequate evidence to currently recommend hydroxyurea treatment

effects. MTD is reached by dose escalation of 5 mg/kg/day every 12 weeks, until neutrophil count falls below 1.5×10^9/l or platelet count below 80×10^9/l. At this point hydroxyurea is interrupted until blood counts recover. It is then restarted at a dose 2.5 mg/kg/day less. In some patients, the counts may already be reduced in pre-treatment steady state, due to causes such as splenomegaly or racial neutropenia. Here, the MTD is difficult to determine and patients should be monitored for a fall in blood counts below steady state. In general we would not recommend exceeding 35 mg/kg/day, the maximum dose used in the MSH study.

An alternative approach to dosing, which has been used in some European centers, is the minimum effective dose, which is determined pragmatically based on the presence or absence of painful crisis symptoms.

For monitoring, full blood count should be taken at 2 and 4 weeks and then monthly. More frequent monitoring should be done after each dose increase. Once on a stable dose, full blood should be checked every 8–10 weeks. Management of myelosuppression is covered in Table 18.2. A modest rise in Hb is often seen with hydroxyurea therapy but excessive rises are may result in hyperviscosity. An increase in Hb of >3 g/l to more than >120 g/l, should be considered an indication for dose reduction or venesection.

Barriers to Wider Prescription

It is reasonable to ask why hydroxyurea is not more widely used in managing SCD. It is the only disease-modifying drug currently licensed, and the evidence of its efficacy, at least in preventing acute vaso-occlusive crises, and improving hematological parameters, is convincing. Some clinicians suggest that there is sufficient evidence now to consider hydroxyurea for all children, even those who are asymptomatic, with the aim of preventing morbidity and mortality in the same way as we would control asthma with bronchodilators and

TABLE 18.2 Management of myelosuppression during hydroxyurea treatment

Neutrophils ($\times 10^9$/L)	Reticulocytes ($\times 10^9$/L)	Hemoglobin (g/l)	Platelets ($\times 10^9$/L)	Hydroxyurea
$\geq 1.5 \times 10^9$/L	$>10 \times 10^9$/L	Within 30 g/l of baseline	$\geq 80 \times 10^9$/L	100 % dose
$<1.5 \times 10^9$/L	$<10 \times 10^9$/L	Fall of >30 g/l from baseline	$<80 \times 10^9$/L	Stop treatment and recheck FBC until hematological recovery. Restart treatment using a dose reduced by 2.5 mg/kg (children) or 500 mg (adults).

anti-inflammatory drugs, or diabetes with insulin or hypoglycemic agents. Using words from a review document produced by the Agency for Healthcare Research and Quality in the US, "The risks of hydroxyurea are acceptable compared with the risks of untreated sickle cell disease".

The approach in the UK and Europe so far has been more conservative, acknowledging these barriers to widespread use of hydroxyurea:

1. Inadequate long-term data on efficacy in preventing chronic complications and improving life expectancy.
2. Inadequate long-term data for reassurance about safety, in particular the risk of infertility in males.
3. Perceptions and misperceptions about toxicities and lack of efficacy of hydroxyurea, sometimes based on anecdotal reports from individuals who have had a negative experience with hydroxyurea
4. Inadequate health care resources for prescribing, monitoring and encouraging adherence.

Clinicians should discuss up-to-date evidence on efficacy and safety of hydroxyurea with their patients and provide written information to allow patients to make an informed choice about whether or not to take hydroxyurea. Sustained adherence to this drug is necessary to ensure clinical benefit, and this will only happen if the patient or parent is convinced that it is in the best interest of the patient to take it.

Blood Transfusion

Blood transfusion has an important role in both the acute and long-term management of SCD. In some acute situations (e.g. acute chest syndrome, acute multi-organ failure, acute anemic episodes in young children) transfusion can be lifesaving and should proceed with minimum delay. In general there have been very few prospective controlled trials to guide transfusion therapy in the acute setting, but several important studies have helped to define the role of chronic transfusion, particularly in primary and secondary prevention of cerebral ischemic damage. Although practice varies, the trend is for increasing use of transfusion, and large centers have seen a rapid increase in patients on planned regular transfusion over the past 10 years. Many patients have had significant clinical benefit from this approach, despite the inconvenience of regular visits to transfusion day care units. Transfusion is becoming better accepted partly because there are more options for control of long-term transfusional iron overload. There are important implications for health care resources as this practice is expanded, and further data on benefits, risks and quality of life are required.

Objective of Transfusion

Although the objectives of transfusion differ in the settings of an acute sickle crisis and long-term primary or secondary prevention, the expected benefits include:

- Correction of anemia
- Improving oxygen carrying capacity of the blood
- Control or reversal of an acute sickling complication
- Control or prevention of chronic vascular or tissue damage

Beneficial Effects of Transfusion

These include:

- Improvement of blood rheology by 'diluting' sickle hemoglobin containing red cells. This effect needs to be balanced against increased blood viscosity if hemoglobin level is too high. The optimal hemoglobin level is about 110 g/l

- Augmentation of oxygen carriage with exogenous hemoglobin
- Temporary suppression of erythropoiesis, and production of HbS-containing red blood cells

Adverse Effects of Transfusion

Transfusion is potentially hazardous in SCD, and some complications are not easy to prevent. The risk/benefit ratio needs to be carefully considered in each case and the patient or parent given a full explanation so that an informed choice can be made. The major risks associated with transfusion in SCD are described below. The safety of transfusion in the UK can be gauged from The Serious Hazards of Transfusion (SHOT) hemovigilance scheme, which encourages reporting of all adverse effects of transfusion, and produces an analysis of these events on an annual basis.

Infection

Since blood is a product derived from human donors, there is a potential risk of inter-human transmission of blood-born infection not clinically manifest in the donor. Chronic viral infections associated with transfusion include hepatitis C virus (HCV), hepatitis B virus (HBV) and human immunodeficiency virus (HIV). Bacterial contamination of red cell units can also result in infection in the recipient. This usually presents as a rapid onset of sepsis and shock during the transfusion. The risk of transfusion-transmitted infection in the UK is extremely low because of the procedures for volunteer donor screening and sensitive serological tests for identifying viral nucleic acid and/or antibody against the virus in donor serum. These are supplemented by rigorous attention to sterile conditions in collection, processing and storage of blood.

There is also a small risk of infection due to emergent infections which are not currently screened for, or for which screening and/or inactivation are not fully effective. An example of this is the prion protein which causes variant Creutzfeld Jacob Disease (vCJD). In the UK, this is thought to be present in the blood donor population, and to have increased as a result of ingestion of beef contaminated with bovine spongiform encephalopathy (BSE) in the 1990s. Four recipients of infected blood have been documented in the UK, three of whom developed vCJD. These infections all occurred in the 1990's, prior to introduction of universal leukodepletion of blood products. Current opinion is that the risk is probably very small and diminishing. Although desirable, there is at present no suitable test for screening blood donations despite.

Alloimmunization

In transfusion practice, red cell allo-immunization usually occurs as a result of transfusion of antigen-positive red cells into an antigen-negative recipient, but can also result from feto-maternal sensitization (most commonly the development of Anti-D in a Rhesus D negative mother). Some alloantibodies appear to develop naturally. The rate of alloimmunization is 18–36 % in SCD patients, which is higher than in a non-sickle population, and increases with donor exposure. Adult patients who were transfused prior to implementation of extended phenotype matching in the 1990's are more likely to be alloimmunized. Some of these have developed multiple alloantibodies and it can be challenging to find compatible blood for them. Since introduction of Rhesus phenotype matching, alloimmunization rates have fallen, and are in the range of 5–15 % of transfused patients.

Alloimmunization can cause a delayed hemolytic transfusion reaction (DHR). This presents as jaundice, fever, chills and fatigue with onset 3–10 days after transfusion. Often this is associated with the onset of an acute painful crisis, or other acute vaso-occlusive event. The patient may be more anemic than prior to the transfusion and serological tests demonstrate a new alloantibody, often with a positive direct antiglobulin test (DAT) indicative of alloantibody-coated recipient red cells. It may be difficult to differentiate between DHR and hemolysis due to an acute pain crisis. Prior to extended phenotype matching, the most frequent alloantibodies were directed against Kell, and Rhesus antigens.

Rhesus allo-immunization stilll occurs, partly due to failures in the provision of rhesus-typed blood (mostly because of miscommunication of the patient's sickle status with the blood bank). The high prevalence of variant rhesus antigens is increasingly recognised as a cause of Rhesus allo-immunization. These result from mutations in the *RHD* and *RHCE* genes. We have observed several cases with poor incremental response to transfusion which have been ascribed to 'auto-anti-e' but are actually anti e Rhesus allantibodies produced in a patient expressing a variant Rhesus e antigen. Other commonly encountered alloantibodies are directed against Duffy (Fy^a, Fy^b or Fy^3), Kidd (Jk^a, Jk^b), S, s and U antigens.

Post-transfusion Hyperhemolysis (PTH)

This is a hemolytic transfusion reaction characterized by destruction of *both* donor and recipient red cells, brisk intravascular hemolysis and life-threatening anemia. The syndrome typically presents 7–10 days after a transfusion, with jaundice, anemia and dark urine (coca-cola coloured) and is often associated with a severe vaso-occlusive crisis. PTH can be difficult to differentiate from DTR. In PTH the hemoglobin level is very low (below the pre-transfusion level), and in contrast to a delayed hemolytic transfusion reaction (DHR), the reticulocyte count may be reduced rather than raised, and the direct antiglobulin test (DAT) is negative. There is often no evidence of a new alloantibody, although this may be demonstrable some time after the initial event. Continuation of transfusion can worsen the hemolysis and should be avoided, unless the patient has life-threatening anemia. Recommended initial treatment is with corticosteroids (methylprednisolone 500 mg iv for 2 days in adults and 10 mg/kg iv for 2 days in children) and intravenous immunoglobulin (1 g/kg for 2 days). When further transfusion cannot be avoided, we usually give intravenous immunoglobulin (1 g/kg for 2 days) and a small volume transfusion after the first infusion of immunoglobulin, together with high dose steroids. It is useful to monitor the colour of the urine, which reverts from dark red to normal colour and is an early sign of resolution of the hemolytic episode.

Procedures for Safe Transfusion in SCD

In view of the increased risks of transfusion in SCD, particularly from alloimmunization and transfusion reactions, it is important that the transfusion laboratory is aware of the diagnosis of SCD and has information about previous transfusion history. Table 18.3 lists the information and tests which are required.

Patients with SCD have special requirements, whether the transfusion is a single episode or part of a long-term transfusion programme. Current recommendations are that blood should be matched against the patient's ABO group, as well as for the Kell (K) and rhesus antigens (C, c, D, E, e). Blood should be sickle negative and, if possible, less than 7 days old. If a patient develops alloantibodies against further red cell antigens then blood needs to be selected which is negative for these antigens.

Indications for Transfusion

These are discussed in the relevant sections and summarized in Tables 18.4 and 18.5. In the context of acute severe anemia and/or progressive sickling, transfusion has a clear role, although the choice between simple and exchange is sometimes not straightforward.

Exchange Transfusion

Advantages and Disadvantages

The main benefits of exchange over simple transfusion are that the sickle hemoglobin percentage can be more rapidly and effectively reduced to target levels (20–30 %) during an acute event without causing a hazardous increase in hematocrit

TABLE 18.3 Procedures for safe transfusion in sickle cell disease

At first visit to clinic	ABO group, antibody screen, full red cell phenotype
	Inform blood transfusion laboratory of the diagnosis of SCD, any previous history of alloimmunization and/or transfusion reactions
	Ensure that special transfusion requirements are flagged on the patient record in the transfusion laboratory
	Check hepatitis B vaccination status and arrange vaccination if not immune
For acute transfusion or planned transfusion (e.g. prior to surgery)	ABO group, antibody screen. Request cross match of required units of blood
	Confirm blood transfusion laboratory aware of diagnosis of SCD and that special transfusion requirements are flagged on the patient record
Initiation and continuation of regular transfusion programme	ABO group, antibody screen. Request cross match of required units of blood
	Confirm blood transfusion laboratory aware of diagnosis of SCD and that special transfusion requirements are flagged on the patient record
	Check hepatitis B vaccination status and arrange vaccination if not immune
	Virus serology: Anti-HIV, anti-HCV, HBsAg, anti-HB core. Virology tests to be repeated annually

and in circulating blood volume. In a chronic exchange programme, removal as well as transfusion of blood can reduce or completely prevent transfusion iron loading, thus avoiding the need for long-term iron chelation therapy. The main drawbacks are extra cost, extra staffing, difficulties with obtaining adequate vascular access, and an increased exposure to red

Table 18.4 Indications for transfusion: Acute complications

Indication	Types of transfusion (simple (S), exchange (E) or not usually indicated (NUI))	Comments
Acute splenic sequestration	S	Top-up to steady state level
Aplastic crisis	S	Top-up to steady state level
Acute painful crisis	NUI	Could potentially worsen the situation through increased blood viscosity. Should be considered if there is an exacerbation of hemolysis (Hb <60 g/l, >20 g/l drop below steady state) or if additional complications are present
Acute chest syndrome (Chap. 6)	S or E	Mild – no transfusion Moderate – simple transfusion Severe – urgent exchange. May need to be preceded by simple transfusion if Hb <70 g/l
Fulminant priapism	S or E	Transfusion indicated (Initially S if Hb <70 g/l) if no resolution with cavernosal aspiration and injection of alpha agonist drug. Exchange transfusion may be indicated prior to surgical shunt procedure
Multi-organ failure	E	Urgent exchange to HbS <30 %. (Initially S IF Hb <70 g/l)

(continued)

TABLE 18.4 (continued)

Indication	Types of transfusion (simple (S), exchange (E) or not usually indicated (NUI))	Comments
Ischemic stroke	E	Urgent exchange to HbS <30 %. (Initially S IF Hb <70 g/l)
Hemorrhagic stroke	S or E	Although there is no direct evidence of benefit, we would recommend optimising Hb to 80 g/l, and consideration of E if surgical or radiological intervention is planned
Girdle syndrome	S or E	If Hb <60 and 20 g/l below baseline, consider simple transfusion E may be indicated in severe episodes
Hepatic sequestration	S	Treat in the same way as acute splenic sequestration
Hepatopathy	E	May be indicated in acute progressive hepatic dysfunction
Retinal artery occlusion	NUI	No evidence of benefit
Overwhelming sepsis	S or E	Transfusion often beneficial if Hb drops (to below 60 g/l or >20 g/l from steady state) or evidence of hypoxemia
Hematuria	S	If Hb drops 20 g/dl below steady state
Acute complications of gallstones	S or E	May be indicated if there is a significant drop in Hb (<60 g/l and 20 g/dl below baseline) or before urgent surgical or endoscopic intervention

Table 18.5 Indications transfusion: primary or secondary prevention

Indication	Level of evidence	Comments
Acute Pain Crisis-prevention	Secondary analysis of RCT data	Should be considered when hydroxyurea is ineffective, refused or contraindicated
Chronic pain	No evidence	Not recommended
Acute ischemic stroke-primary prevention	RCT	Recommended in children with confirmed abnormal TCD
Acute ischemic stroke-secondary prevention	RCT	RCT evidence that transfusion and chelation is more effective than hydroxyurea and venesection in children. Recommended in children and adults. See Chap. 7
Silent cerebral ischemia	RCT	May reduce risk of ischemic stroke and progression in children with SCI
Cerebral vasculopathy	Expert opinion/ case series	May stabilize or improve stenotic lesions in children. No evidence of improvement in moyamoya
Acute hemorrhagic stroke-primary or secondary prevention	Expert opinion/ case series	Not generally recommended
Prevention of recurrent ACS	Secondary analysis of RCT data	Should be considered when hydroxyurea is ineffective, refused or contraindicated

(continued)

TABLE 18.5 (continued)

Indication	Level of evidence	Comments
Chronic sickle lung syndrome	Expert opinion/ case series	May be considered on an individual basis in symptomatic patients with hypoxemia, and progressive pulmonary damage
Pulmonary hypertension	Expert opinion/ case series	May be considered on an individual basis in patients with symptoms of PHT and TR jet velocity >3 m/sec after evaluation in specialist PHT clinic.
Chronic renal failure	Expert opinion/ case series	Indicated for severe anemia where erythropoietin is ineffective
Priapism	Expert opinion/ case series	Effective in preventing recurrent episodes of severe stuttering or fulminant priapism in some patients when drug therapy and hydroxyurea are not effective or not acceptable
Retinopathy: prevention of complications of proliferative retinopathy and retinal artery occlusion	No evidence	Not recommended
Chronic liver disease (hepatopathy)	Expert opinion/ case series	May reduce risk of progression

Acute splenic sequestration-prevention of recurrent episodes	Expert opinion/case series	Reduces risk of recurrence to enable delay of splenectomy until age 5
Avascular necrosis	Secondary analysis of RCT	In pre-pubertal children, may be helpful in prevention, and possibly remodelling of affected hip
Lower limb ulceration	Expert opinion/case series	May be considered in cases of refractory ulceration. Simple transfusion if Hb <60 g/l
Growth failure and pubertal failure	Expert opinion/case series	Can be helpful in accelerating pubertal growth in severely anemic children
Elective surgery	RCT	Simple transfusion in HbSS patients with moderate or low risk surgery and Hb <90 g/l. Exchange if high risk surgery or Hb >90 g/l and moderate/low risk surgery. See Chap. 16
Pregnancy	RCT	Routine prophylactic transfusion not indicated in all patients, but used in selected patients with recurrent acute pain crisis. Transfuse to treat acute complications during pregnancy

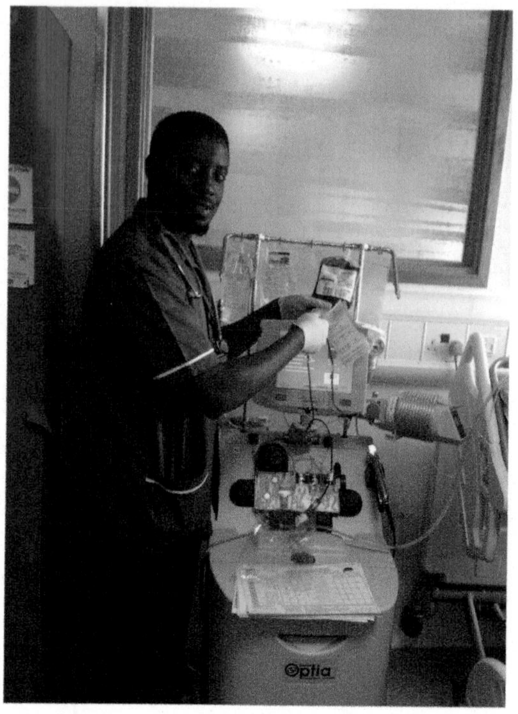

FIGURE 18.2 Erythrocytapheresis in progress

cell donor units which may increase the risks of alloimmunization and transfusion-transmitted infection.

Exchange transfusion can be done manually, or using automated erythrocytapheresis (Fig. 18.2). In practice the apheresis equipment and technical skills necessary for automated exchange are generally restricted to large regional sickle cell units.

Vascular Access

Children and adults with SCD generally have poor peripheral venous access, and it is often necessary to insert a temporary large-bore central venous catheter (subclavian, internal jugular or femoral) to perform an emergency exchange transfusion.

For younger children managed on a high dependency unit, an arterial line often works well. Some patients have adequate peripheral venous access to sustain long-term exchange transfusion via peripheral veins, but the majority require either temporary or long-term central venous access. Many adult patients on long-term exchange transfusion have a temporary central line (usually femoral) inserted under ultrasound guidance and then removed at the end of the exchange procedure. An alternative is a single or double lumen Port-a cath (Figs. 18.3 and 18.4), which requires insertion by a surgeon or interventional radiologist. These devices carry a significant risk of thrombosis and infection, and there is a high rate of removal and replacement. It is important to restrict their use to experienced staff, to insist on aseptic procedures and manage potential infection or blockage promptly.

Practical Aspects of Exchange Transfusion

The aims of the procedure are:

- To ensure that hemoglobin level remains in the range 80–10 g/dl and does not exceed 110 g/l
- To ensure that the entire process is isovolumetric
- To decrease HbS to <30 %

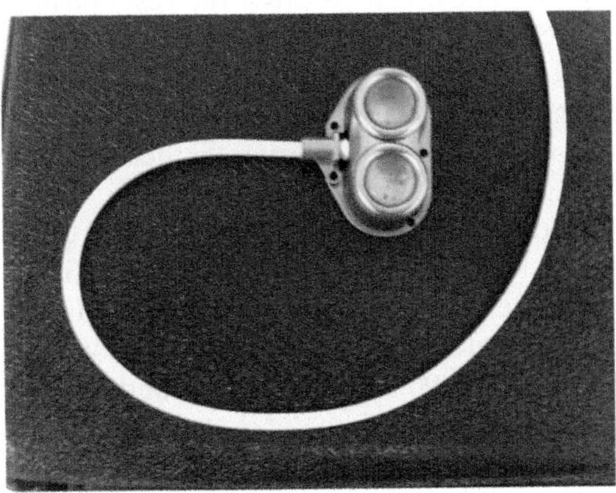

FIGURE 18.3 Double lumen portacath used for exchange transfusion

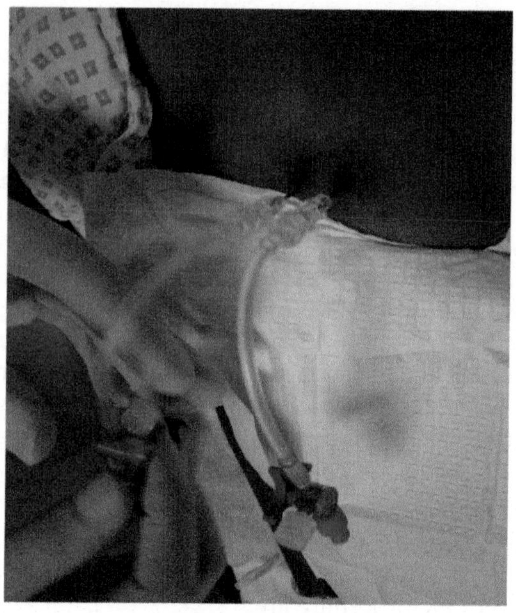

FIGURE 18.4 Double lumen portacath being accessed during erythrocytophereis

It is unsafe to initiate an exchange transfusion if the hemoglobin level is very low, as is often the case during an acute severe sickle cell crisis. If the starting hemoglobin level is significantly less than the steady state value, or below 70 g/l, the exchange transfusion should be preceded with a top-up transfusion of 10–20 ml/kg to bring the hemoglobin level up to about 90 g/l.

In order to calculate of amount of blood to remove and to transfuse, it is best to think in terms of hematocrit rather than hemoglobin level: The hematocrit of plasma-reduced red cells in the UK is about 0.6. If the patient's hematocrit is 0.3 (corresponding to about 90 g/l hemoglobin), and the haematocrit is to be maintained, the volume of red cells to transfuse is half the volume of blood venesected from the patient. The remaining volume for replacement should be crystalloid fluid. The volume of the full exchange required to bring the HbS percentage to below 30 % is usually 60–80 ml/kg, rather less if the patient has already had a simple transfusion. Our protocol for manual exchange transfusion is shown in Appendix 4.

In the case of automated exchange, the volumes are calculated by the built-in software on the apparatus. The advantage of automated exchange is that it is a relatively quick procedure taking only two hours in comparison with 4–6 hours for a manual procedure. It will often produce a lower final HbS% than a manual exchange and is associated with less iron overload. The decision about using manual or automated exchange will usually depend on the availability of staff and equipment rather than clinical indications. Even in specialist units where equipment is available, trained staff are not always at hand outside of working hours to perform automated exchanges.

Training in exchange transfusion should be included in the education of hematology staff and specialist nurses. Junior hematology doctors should be able to perform a manual red cell exchange procedure supported by a haematologist or nurse specialist.

Iron Overload and Its Management

Iron overload in SCD is predominantly a consequence of transfusion. Patients who have not been transfused, or only transfused on rare occasions are not significantly iron loaded, and may even become iron deficient. This contrasts with thalassemia major (TM), where iron accumulates even in non-transfusion dependent patients as a result of increased gastro-intestinal iron absorption.

The time course of iron loading also differs. Children with thalassemia major (TM) usually start transfusions in the first year of life, whereas for SCD children it is usually between the age of 2 and 9 years. Iron overload in older patients can be very significant even in those who have only been transfused intermittently over the years.

Less is known about the long-term clinical complications of transfusion iron overload in SCD than for patients with TM. Hepatic iron loading develops rapidly, but it is not yet clear how this impacts on long-term morbidity and mortality. Liver biopsies in children on chronic transfusion programmes usually show absent or only mild fibrotic changes, despite high liver iron levels. However, chronic liver disease in older patients is an important cause of morbidity and mortality, and transfusional iron overload is probably an important co-factor in disease progression (Chap. 13) SCD patients are relatively protected against myocardial iron overload and iron-related endocrine complications compared to TM. This may be related to increased hepcidin production stimulated by hemolysis and chronic inflammation. Hepcidin prevents iron export from reticuloendothelial stores and reduces the plasma pool of labile iron which is available for uptake into target organs.

Assessment of Iron Overload

A combination of methods is needed for accurate assessment of transfusion iron loading and response to treatment.

Net Volume of Blood Infused Per Year (ml/kg Red Cells)

Net transfused volume of red cells should be systematically recorded at each transfusion visit, and the total calculated at the end of the year. For a child on a chronic simple transfusion programme, transfusion volume is usually in the range 100–175 ml/kg/year (60–100 ml/kg of red cells), equating to a daily rate of iron loading of about 0.2–0.4 mg/kg/day.

Serum Ferritin (SF)

SF levels are harder to interpret than in TM. There are several reasons for this: An association between high SF and adverse clinical outcomes has not yet been established as it has in TM, high SF levels may be related to acute crises or chronic inflammation rather than iron overload, and the correlation between SF and liver iron levels is poor. Nevertheless, trends in SF do reflect changes in liver iron concentration over time. We recommend that SF levels are measured 3 monthly to monitor the trend and annual average level should be recorded. Levels should ideally be maintained in the region 500–1,500 ug/l.

Liver Iron Concentration (LIC) by MRI (R2 Ferriscan® or T2*)

This is the method of choice for assessment of body iron stores, and sequential scans done on an annual basis provide an excellent means of monitoring results of chelation therapy and adjusting dosing. There have been problems with the calibration of LIC measured by T2* MRI in the UK, and most services now use Ferriscan®, which is commercially available and has more robust standardization. MR sequences are analysed and reported centrally. We recommend that LIC is maintained in the range 2–7 mg/g dry weight.

Control of Transfusional Iron Overload

Sequential Phlebotomy

If a decision has already been taken to discontinue transfusion, this is an effective means of reducing body iron stores. Monthly phlebotomies (5 ml/kg body weight if Hb 70–80 g/l or 10 ml/kg body weight if Hb >80 g/l) are safe in patients who do not have severe cardiorespiratory disease. This is particularly suitable for adult or adolescent patients who have been switched to hydroxyurea. The SWiTCH trial did not demonstrate better control of iron stores with this approach compared to transfusion and chelation, but this was probably because there was a prolonged overlap of transfusion and hydroxyurea before phlebotomy was instituted.

Regular Exchange Transfusion

This is described in the previous section. Both automated and manual exchange transfusion programmes can be designed to ensure that there is no net iron loading during each exchange procedure. If the patient is already iron loaded, iron chelation therapy is usually required until iron stores have reduced to safe levels. Since there is no net iron loading, the chelation regime can often be reduced in intensity to minimise adverse effects.

Iron Chelation Therapy

Most young children initiated on long-term transfusion are not suitable for regular exchange transfusion, and during the first few years of regular transfusion accumulate a significant amount of iron. We recommend iron chelation therapy is started after 1 year, when they have received about 10–12 transfusions. By this stage, SF is generally in excess of 1,000 ug/l. Most studies show that chelation is less effective in SCD than in TM patients. This may be due to sub-optimal adherence to treatment, increased side effects leading to frequent dose interruptions, or impaired chelator efficacy. Regular monitoring for efficacy and adverse effects is crucial. After starting therapy, 3 monthly dose escalations are usually necessary to maximise efficacy. Quite often, temporary dose reductions are necessary because of adverse effects. The dose also needs to be adjusted as the child's weight increases.

Monitoring and encouraging adherence to medication is vital. We suggest that this is done every month when they attend for transfusion, as well as through home visits by community nurse specialists. Problems with adherence may be due to intolerance (especially in the case of regular subcutaneous injections of desferrioxamine), side effects (particularly gastro-intestinal intolerance in the case of deferasirox), and lack of motivation. One of the important roles of the nurse specialist is to explore ways of improving adherence.

Two iron chelating drugs are currently licensed for iron chelation in SCD:

Desferrioxamine (DFO) needs to be given by subcutaneous infusion over 8–12 h five to six times per week. Although this is a demanding regime, chelation results can be excellent if adequate adherence can be ensured and this option should be considered for motivated children and parents. The main side effects in growing children include damage to the growth plates of the long bones and spine, hearing loss and retinopathy. These side effects can be avoided if the dose is kept in the range 20–40 mg/kg. This is particularly important in patients with low iron stores (SF < 1,000 and LIC <5 mg/g dw).

Deferasirox (DFX) is a once daily oral agent which requires dispersal in water, orange or apple juice. We would consider DFX the chelator of choice for SCD patients, and provided the dose can be escalated into the range 30–35 mg/kg/day, SF and LIC levels can be brought down and maintained in the acceptable range in most cases. With regards to side effects, data so far suggest that DFX has an acceptable safety profile, provided that regular clinical and biochemical monitoring is done. The commonest side effects reported are gastrointestinal symptoms, skin rash, transient increases in serum creatinine and transaminitis.

Deferiprone (DFP) is currently only licensed in TM, but it has also been used in SCD patients who have not been able to tolerate the licensed agents. There are currently trials underway to compare DFP with DFO and with DFX in SCD patients. The main side effects of DFP are agranulocytosis (in about 1 %) and arthropathy.

Hemopoietic Stem Cell Transplantation (HSCT)

HSCT in Children

Hemopoietic stem cell transplantation (HSCT) is currently the only curative option for SCD. To date, about 1,200 transplants have been reported in the European and US transplant registries, the majority in children with an HLA matched sibling donor. Using a matched sibling donor and a myeloablative regime, the rates for mortality, rejection, and cure are 5 %, 5 % and 90 % respectively. After successful HSCT, acute vaso-occlusive crises are abolished, CNS disease stabilized (but usually not improved), TCD flow normalized and quality of life is generally much improved. Long-term complications of HSCT in children include loss of fertility due to primary gonadal failure, skeletal complications (osteoporosis) and a very small increase in the risk of malignant disease. The long-term outcome is generally much in favour of BMT compared to standard care.

Indications for HSCT

Current indications for matched sibling HSCT in children in the UK are listed in Table 18.6.

Elsewhere in Europe and N America, the indications are often more liberal and some specialists advocate HSCT for

TABLE 18.6 Current indications for matched sibling HSCT in children as recommended by the British Bone Marrow Transplant Society

Recurrent vaso-occlusive complications (acute pain or acute chest syndrome) not responding to hydroxyurea
Past history of ischaemic stroke and/or severe cerebral vasculopathy
Abnormal Transcranial Doppler flow with evidence of ischaemic cerebral damage
Severe avascular necrosis
Multiple red cell alloantibodies restricting availability of blood for transfusion
Nephropathy
Problems relating to future care (e.g. likely return to home country where health care services are inadequate)

any child with HbSS, irrespective of severity, if an HLA compatible sibling donor is available.

Risks and Benefits

Most specialists begin the discussion about possible HSCT with parents early during the first year of life, and then at appropriate occasions later in childhood. The first outcome of this discussion is an agreement for compatibility testing of siblings (if available). If a donor is identified, a fuller discussion and assessment is initiated, together with referral to a specialist transplant unit. The decision to go ahead can be very difficult for parents, partly because it is difficult to predict long-term prognosis for a young child who may not be particularly severely affected at the time of the discussion.

The Transplant Procedure

HSCT in SCD should only be performed in centers experienced in transplanting hemoglobinopathy patients. The technical and practical details of transplant procedures are beyond the scope of this book. Protocols have evolved and are becoming tailored to the particular features of SCD. Acute graft versus host disease appears to be increased with use of peripheral blood, and bone marrow is advised as a source of donor stem cells. Furthermore, there is a higher risk of delayed engraftment with umbilical cord blood transplants, and cord blood is generally not recommended as the sole source of stem cells, at least in older children. There are specific requirements for conditioning in SCD transplants, including pre-transplant hypertransfusion and marrow suppression with hydroxyurea. Granulocyte colony stimulating factor is not used for stimulation of neutrophil recovery, because of the risk of precipitating a severe vaso-occlusive crisis. In the first days and weeks after the transplant, in addition to a higher risk of acute neurological events in the presence of cerebral vasculopathy, there is also a significant increased risk of PRES.

Alternative Donors

Unfortunately only 10–15 % of patients have an HLA matched sibling donor. Alternatives include matched unrelated donors, or haplo-identical (half-matched) family donors. In general, mortality and morbidity are increased with use of alternative donors and these transplants should only be considered in patients with severe complications of SCD who are deteriorating in spite of optimal standard therapy (blood transfusion or hydroxyurea). They should only be undertaken as part of a research protocol.

Use of well-matched unrelated donors is limited by the lack of volunteers from black ethnic groups on the international HSCT donor registries. Currently the probability of finding a donor is <15 %. Haplo-HSCT using a parent or sibling is attractive because almost all patients will have a donor. It is currently being evaluated in children and adults with severe complications of SCD (e.g. progressive neurovascular complications despite optimal transfusion), using non-myeloablative conditioning with sustained immunosuppressive regimes designed to maintain a stable mixed chimeric state, and to prevent graft- versus- host disease. Current experience indicates that stable engraftment is possible with low risk of graft versus host disease. Unfortunately, the graft failure rate is over 50 %, which is unacceptable, and protocol modifications will be necessary to improve engraftment. Accumulation of pooled experience over the next few years will better define the role of haplo BMT.

HSCT in Adults

The outcomes for adults using HLA-matched sibling donors are poorer than in children. However, a recent single-center study using non-myeloablative conditioning and a novel immunosuppressive regime has reported long-term stable mixed donor-recipient chimerism (donor and host cells co-existing) in nine out of ten patients. A follow-up on this report confirmed these results in a larger number of patients and showed that some patients maintained full engraftment after withdrawal of immunosuppression. The indications for transplant included irreversible end-organ damage, stroke or other significant CNS events. Interestingly some of the patients had severe acute and chronic pain, which gradually resolved enabling withdrawal of chronic opioid medication. These results are encouraging and need to be replicated in other centers. Unfortunately, the requirement for an HLA-matched sibling donor still restricts this approach to a small minority of adult patients. There will, however, be a population of adults who were never offered HSCT during childhood and may not realise they have a suitable donor.

There is very little evidence about outcome of HSCT in adults using alternative donors and at the current time these should only be performed as part of a research protocol.

Umbilical Cord Blood HSCT and Storage of Cord Blood

Umbilical cord blood from babies who are known to be HLA-matched with an affected sibling can be stored and used as a source of hematopoietic stem cells. This scenario would usually occur after pre-natal diagnosis (PND) has confirmed that the sibling is unaffected, and subsequent HLA-typing of the CVS sample has confirmed HLA matching. It is important to inform parents of this option in the early stages of pregnancy after they have decided to undergo PND. Sometimes parents request storage of cord blood, without PND being done. In this situation, without knowledge of the SCD status or HLA compatibility of the fetus, cord banking would probably not be funded by health authorities.

Gene Therapy

Gene therapy is an exciting prospect for cure or control of SCD in the future, but is not yet a treatment option in the clinic. Despite decades of research into the molecular genetics of haemoglobin disorders, control of gene expression and potential gene therapy technology, there are still significant challenges concerning the efficacy and safety of this approach. Up until recently, the focus has been on thalassaemia, and currently there are at least two Phase 1 trials of potential gene therapy protocols for thalassaemia major or intermedia. The approach involves preparation of an engineered lentivirus vector containing the coding portion of the beta globin gene together with the important regulatory elements which drive high levels of gene expression in the environment of the developing erythroblast. The vector construct is used to infect haematopoietic stem cells from the patient, and the lentivirus-encoded genes control integration of the engineered beta globin gene into the DNA of the host cell. A large number of treated host cells are then reinfused into the patient. In order for the manipulated stem cells to populate the marrow, some pre-treatment to suppress the bone marrow and immume system of the patient is needed. Animal studies have shown successful gene transfer in mouse models of β thalassemia. There has been a recent report of successful gene transfer in one patient with haemoglobin E β thalassaemia who has subsequently expressed the normal β globin gene and become transfusion independent.

Alternative approaches to gene therapy, for instance by 'gene correction' using engineered zinc finger endonucleases to recognise and correct the specific sickle cell mutation in the beta globin gene, or disrupt the genetic control of fetal haemoglobin suppression, to enable resumption of high levels of expression are in earlier stages of development.

Concluding Remarks

From the above, it is apparent that the clinician has limited options for treatment of SCD, and a fairly thin evidence base from clinical trials to guide decisions. Currently, one of the most difficult decisions is whether to offer any treatment at all, particularly to patients who are asymptomatic or have mild, intermittent symptoms and a reasonable quality of life.

Bibliography

Bolton-Maggs P, Poles D, Watt A, et al. The Annual SHOT Report 2012. Available at http://www.shotuk.org/wp-content/uploads/2013/08/SHOT-Annual-Report-2012.pdf.

Brawley OW, Cornelius LJ, Edwards LR, et al. National Institutes of Health Consensus Development Conference Statement: Hydroxyurea Treatment for Sickle Cell Disease. Ann Intern Med. 2008;148(12):932–8.

Charache S, Terrin ML, Moore RD, et al. Effect of hydroxyurea on the frequency of painful crises in sickle cell anemia. Investigators of the Multicenter Study of Hydroxyurea in Sickle Cell Anemia. N Engl J Med. 1995;332:1317–22.

Hsieh MM, Kang EM, Fitzhugh CD, et al. Allogeneic hematopoietic stem-cell transplantation for sickle cell disease. N Engl J Med. 2009;361:2309–17.

Lanzkron S, Strouse JJ, Wilson R, et al. Systematic Review: Hydroxyurea for the Treatment of Adults with Sickle Cell Disease. Ann Intern Med. 2008;148:939–55.

Liebelt EL, Balk SJ, Faber W, et al. Expert Panel Report. NTP-CERHR Expert Panel Report on the Reproductive and Developmental Toxicity of Hydroxyurea. Birth Defects Research (Part B). 2007;80:259–366.

Lobo CL, Pinto JF, Nascimento EM. The effect of hydroxycarbamide therapy on survival of children with sickle cell disease. Br J Hematol. 2013;161(6):852–60.

Locatelli F, Pagliara D. Allogeneic Hematopietic Stem Cell Transplantation in Children with Sickle Cell Disease. Pediatr Blood Cancer. 2012;59:372–6.

Milkins C, Berryman J, Cantwell C, et al. Guidelines for pre-transfusion compatibility procedures in blood transfusion laboratories. Transfus Med. 2013;23(1):3–35.

Steinberg MH, McCarthy WF, Castro O, et al. The risks and benefits of long-term use of hydroxyurea in sickle cell anemia: A 17.5 year follow-up. Am J Hematol. 2010;85:403–8.

Voskaridou E, Christoulas D, Bilalis A, et al. The effects of prolonged administration of hydroxyurea on morbidity and mortality in adult patients with sickle cell syndromes: results of a 17 year single-center trial (LaSHS). Blood. 2010;115(12):2354–63.

Wang WC, Ware RE, Miller ST, et al. Hydroxycarbamide in very young children with sickle-cell anemia: a multicenter, randomized, controlled trial (BABY HUG). Lancet. 2011;377:1663–72.

Chapter 19
Out-Patient Management

Pediatric Aspects

Overview

Children with HbSS should be seen routinely every 3 months up to the age of 2 years, and then 6 monthly. Children with HbSC can be seen every 6 months and then annually from age 5. The visit following each birthday should be scheduled as an annual review. Many clinics have developed out-patient proformas to allow a systematic annual evaluation of the child, to assess severity and to evaluate parameters which may be of prognostic value in the long-term. Measurements of height, weight and pubertal development are essential for assessing and comparing growth and development. Blood pressure, urinalysis and oxygen saturation may be predictive of long-term complications. Steady state blood parameters (including full blood count, reticulocyte count, renal function, percentage HbF and lactate dehydrogenase) have important prognostic and clinical value and should be assessed annually.

It is important to assess the parent/carer's ability to provide care and support for the child. This depends on socioeconomic factors as well as on the level of engagement and understanding about the condition. In some cases, there is a persistent denial of the condition and an unwillingness to

J. Howard, P. Telfer, *Sickle Cell Disease in Clinical Practice*, In Clinical Practice, DOI 10.1007/978-1-4471-2473-3_19,

divulge the diagnosis even to close family members. Erratic adherence to prophylactic medication (especially oral penicillin) irregular attendance at out-patient visits, a tendency to under-estimate the significance of the condition and failure to attend hospital or to call the community nurse specialist during a significant acute illness are disturbing signs.

Other Common Pediatric Out-Patient Problems

Some of the common chronic problems often highlighted during out-patient visits are listed below. Management is challenging and general pediatric protocols are often poorly effective.

- Fatigue
- Headaches
- Nocturnal enuresis
- Pica
- Persisting jaundice
- Poor growth and delayed puberty

Schooling Issues

Schooling is a significant challenge for more severely affected children. Factors which prevent the child reaching their potential include:

- Poor school attendance due to illness and clinic appointments
- Lack of engagement in class activities due to fatigue and/or pain
- Difficulty with engagement in gymnastics and sports due to fatigue and tendency of physical activity to provoke crises

A child will not reach their academic potential at school if experiencing frequent painful crises, and good out-patient control of sickle pain is essential. Minor crises can be managed at school, with time out in a quiet place for rest and supervized simple analgesia. It is not always necessary for the parent to be called to take the child home. Minimising the effort and fatigue in actually getting to and from school, and an agreement for restriction of outdoor activities are all important. The ability to undertake sports and gym activities is variable and needs to be assessed on an individual basis. Severely affected children get fatigued with moderate exertion. Being forced to engage in outdoor sports is a potent stimulus to crisis in many SCD children.

For children with stroke or silent infarct it is helpful to make a psychometric assessment of cognitive deficits. This will help in requesting and planning a Statement of Special Educational Needs. Simple inputs in class can be very helpful. For those with concentration/attention and processing difficulties, sitting near the front of the class, allowing more time for tasks, and training to break complex tasks down into easier steps can improve performance and attainment.

It is essential to develop good communication with school teachers, school health services, and the Special Educational Needs Co-ordinator. The aim is to develop a school care plan for each child which is drawn up and regularly reviewed by the school nurse, drawing on the support of the SCD multidisciplinary team.

Adult Aspects

Adults with HbSS should be reviewed at least six monthly and those with HbSC and HbS β thalassemia at least once a year. For those managed jointly by a specialist and local center, the annual review should be done at the specialist centre.

Employment and Higher Education

School leavers with SCD are expected to enter higher education or employment. It is important that they continue to engage with SCD services and are directed to services local to where they are studying or working. Young people should be asked about further education plans during outpatient consultations and if they are moving away for study a referral to the local service should be made so that there is no gap in care. This is particularly important for patients on a chronic transfusion program or hydroxyurea. The individual acute pain management plan should be shared with the new center so that plans can be put in place in advance of their attending with an acute painful crisis.

Genetic Counselling

A frequent reminder about the pattern of inheritance of SCD is good practice when seeing adolescents and adults. New partners should be offered genetic testing so that the couple are aware of their risk and of the options available to them if the partner is found to be a carrier.

Contraception

Contraception should be discussed with patients as part of their routine care. Barrier methods are safe and effective in women with SCD. Progestogen containing contraceptives are also safe and effective and there is some evidence that these may be associated with a decrease in painful episodes. The UK Medical Eligibility Criteria (UKMEC) advise that the progestogen only pill, Depo-Provera, Levonorgestrel IUDs (Mirena) and emergency contraception can be used safely in all clinical situations. Implantable progestogens should be included in this group. The combined oral contraceptive pill and the copper intrauterine device are associated with some clinical risk, but in most clinical circumstances their use would be justifiable. They can be recommended if a safer alternative cannot be used.

Other Health Issues

Patients may have other chronic inflammatory conditions which adversely affect SCD. Co-ordinated care requires good communication and formulation of a joint care plan which take into account the interactions between the conditions. Examples of these include systemic lupus erythematosis (SLE), sarcoidosis and ulcerative colitis.

Care of the Older Patient

As survival improves we are seeing increased numbers of older patients (over 60 years). These patients are not only more likely to have chronic complications of SCD, but are also more likely to have other co-existent health problems. They need careful monitoring and management of these complications.

Transition

Transition is the purposeful planned movement of adolescents with chronic diseases from child-centered to adult-centered health care systems and encompasses the process of psychosocial evolution from adolescent to adult. Transition poses particular challenges for all young people with chronic diseases with regard to self-awareness and autonomy. The aims of the transition process are to enable the adolescent to develop an understanding and acceptance of the condition and also to develop a psychology and lifestyle which will have a positive impact on their long-term health and wellbeing. Parents and carers may have concerns about the young person's ability for self care after the loss of support of the pediatric team. There are also understandable concerns about moving inpatient care to an adult ward setting, where most of the patients are elderly and the ward nurses are fewer in number. Some hospitals have adolescent units, and these generally provide a more appropriate environment for managing teenagers and young adults with acute complications. Adolescents with SCD may be relatively immature physically and emotionally, and lack the independence needed to access health care in the adult environment. Starting the transition process early and ensuring good communication between the adult and pediatric team are crucial.

Transition can be enhanced by establishing a transitional team, who are responsible for co-ordinating pediatric and adult input and helping to guide the patient through the process. Transition clinics, where the pediatric and adult teams see the patient together to hand over care, are widely used. Another helpful initiative is a 'Transition Day' where young people are introduced to the adult service, meet patients who have already transitioned and have the opportunity to network. Some units have used a transition passport which the young person and care giver complete together.

New Patients

It is not uncommon for patients to transfer from one clinic to another. This may be because they have moved home, started university or relocated for new employment. Patients previously living in other countries or continents (particularly Africa) may be referred into specialized services, after registering with a local family doctor. On registration in the SCD clinic, a full medical history is required including a description of previous hospital admissions, blood transfusions, operations and chronic disease complications. A detailed baseline physical examination should also be done.

Investigations include confirmation of the diagnosis of SCD, G6PD status, full red cell phenotype, Hepatitis B and C and HIV status as well as the baseline blood tests recommended in Table 4.1. Screening tests, such as echocardiography and evaluation of urinary protein should be discussed and ordered if results are not up to date.

The new patient should be introduced to the multidisciplinary team, shown round the department and given verbal and written information about how to make contact with the service and how to access emergency care. This is a good opportunity for discussing their usual analgesic regimes, both as outpatients and when in hospital.

Annual Review

We regard the annual review as pivotal in the organization of long-term care. For patients of all genotypes, this is an opportunity for a holistic review of medical, psychological and social needs. It works particularly well as a one-stop multidisciplinary clinic. These might include consultations with the nurse specialist, psychologist, dietician, dentist, ophthalmologist and transcranial Doppler sonographer.

The annual review allows a systematic assessment of the patient, an appraisal of their understanding of the condition and their specific needs. It also provides a framework for systematic recording of clinical data which can be shared between local and specialist centers. This data can potentially be fed into a national register. An example is the UK National Hemoglobinopathy Registry, which is set up to enable annual review data to be entered 'real-time' provided the patient has previously consented for entry on the register.

The annual review also offers an opportunity to discuss disease modifying therapy, new medications, research findings, ongoing research studies and reproductive choices.

If there are new clinical findings suggestive of a chronic complication, referral to specialist clinics may be appropriate.

An example of an annual review proforma can be found in Appendix 5.

Bibliography

Howard J, Woodhead T, Musumadi L, et al. Moving young people with sickle cell disease from pediatric to adult services. Br J Hosp Med (London). 2010;71(6):310–4.

Appendix 1: Proforma for Pain Assessment

Patients Name: Hosp #

Sex M / F (circle) DOB

PAIN AND ANALGESIA ASSESSMENT

Date/Time

Site of pain:

Duration of pain:

Description of pain:

- Sharp ☐
- Burning ☐
- Throbbing ☐
- Shooting ☐
- Aching ☐
- Stabbing ☐
- Sore ☐
- Crushing ☐
- Other ☐

Precipitant/Triggers:

- Infection ☐
- Dehydration ☐
- Cold weather ☐
- Hot weather ☐
- Stress ☐
- Physical activity ☐
- Other ☐

Analgesia taken in the last 8 hrs:..

Patients with **ANY** of the below should be referred for medical review

- Chest pain, Shortness of breath, Hypoxia (oxygen saturations <94%)
- Fever/rigors (Temp >38°C), Hypotension (BP <90/60)
- Tachycardia > 100 (even after pain has settled following analgesia)
- Raised respiratory rate of > 20 (even after pain has settled following analgesia)
- New neurological symptoms, headache, confusion, numbness of limbs
- Abdominal pains
- Priapism (persistent erection)
- Pregnancy
- Visual loss or bleeding in the eye
- PAR > four
- Concerns from the nursing team about the patient's clinical condition

J. Howard, P. Telfer, *Sickle Cell Disease in Clinical Practice*, In Clinical Practice, DOI 10.1007/978-1-4471-2473-3,

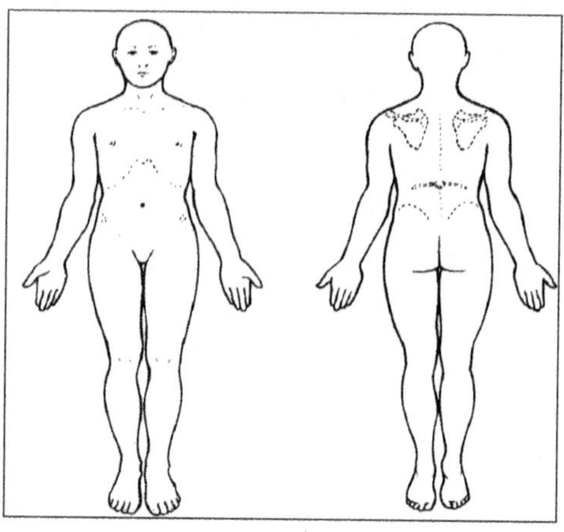

MARK SITE OF PATIENT'S PAIN ABOVE

ASSESSMENTS

Notes

Time of 1st dose analgesia: **List of drugs given in the Day Unit:**

(Re-assess pain after 30mins)

2nd Assessment:

Appendix 2: Examples of Analgesia Protocols

(i) Example of an adult analgesia protocol using subcuteneous morphine given by infusion pump as patient controlled analgesia

Morphine Sulphate 50 ml pre-filled syringe
100 mg/50 ml = 2 mg/ml

Background infusion rate	1 mg/h
Lockout time	5 min
Bolus	1 mg (0.5 ml)
	This may be escalated to 1.5–2 mg if clinically indicated
Dose duration	1 min
Dose limit	4 h limit = 40 mg

J. Howard, P. Telfer, *Sickle Cell Disease in Clinical Practice*, In Clinical Practice, DOI 10.1007/978-1-4471-2473-3,

(ii) Example of a pediatric acute analgesia protocol

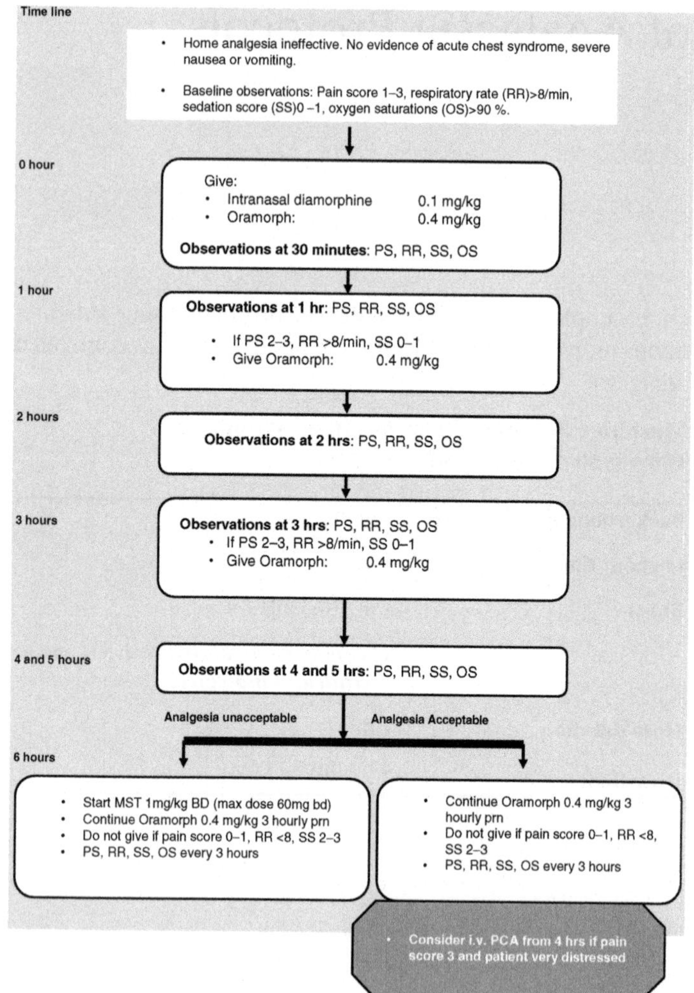

Appendix 3: Pain Assessment Scale

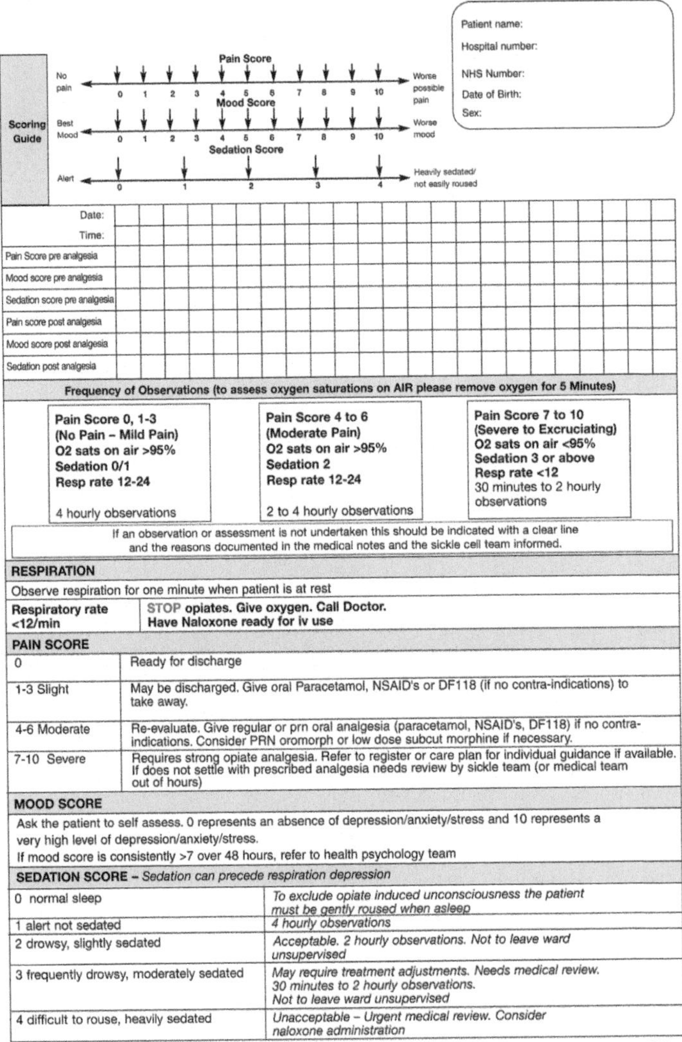

Date:																							
Time:																							
Pain Score pre analgesia																							
Mood score pre analgesia																							
Sedation score pre analgesia																							
Pain score post analgesia																							
Mood score post analgesia																							
Sedation post analgesia																							

Frequency of Observations (to assess oxygen saturations on AIR please remove oxygen for 5 Minutes)

Pain Score 0, 1-3 **(No Pain – Mild Pain)** **O2 sats on air >95%** **Sedation 0/1** **Resp rate 12-24** 4 hourly observations	**Pain Score 4 to 6** **(Moderate Pain)** **O2 sats on air >95%** **Sedation 2** **Resp rate 12-24** 2 to 4 hourly observations	**Pain Score 7 to 10** **(Severe to Excruciating)** **O2 sats on air <95%** **Sedation 3 or above** **Resp rate <12** 30 minutes to 2 hourly observations

If an observation or assessment is not undertaken this should be indicated with a clear line and the reasons documented in the medical notes and the sickle cell team informed.

RESPIRATION	
Observe respiration for one minute when patient is at rest	
Respiratory rate <12/min	**STOP opiates. Give oxygen. Call Doctor. Have Naloxone ready for iv use**

PAIN SCORE	
0	Ready for discharge
1-3 Slight	May be discharged. Give oral Paracetamol, NSAID's or DF118 (if no contra-indications) to take away.
4-6 Moderate	Re-evaluate. Give regular or prn oral analgesia (paracetamol, NSAID's, DF118) if no contra-indications. Consider PRN oromorph or low dose subcut morphine if necessary.
7-10 Severe	Requires strong opiate analgesia. Refer to register or care plan for individual guidance if available. If does not settle with prescribed analgesia needs review by sickle team (or medical team out of hours)

MOOD SCORE

Ask the patient to self assess. 0 represents an absence of depression/anxiety/stress and 10 represents a very high level of depression/anxiety/stress.
If mood score is consistently >7 over 48 hours, refer to health psychology team

SEDATION SCORE – *Sedation can precede respiration depression*	
0 normal sleep	*To exclude opiate induced unconsciousness the patient must be gently roused when asleep*
1 alert not sedated	*4 hourly observations*
2 drowsy, slightly sedated	*Acceptable. 2 hourly observations. Not to leave ward unsupervised*
3 frequently drowsy, moderately sedated	*May require treatment adjustments. Needs medical review. 30 minutes to 2 hourly observations. Not to leave ward unsupervised*
4 difficult to rouse, heavily sedated	*Unacceptable – Urgent medical review. Consider naloxone administration*

07/09

J. Howard, P. Telfer, *Sickle Cell Disease in Clinical Practice*, In Clinical Practice, DOI 10.1007/978-1-4471-2473-3,

Appendix 4: Manual Exchange Transfusion

Paediatric

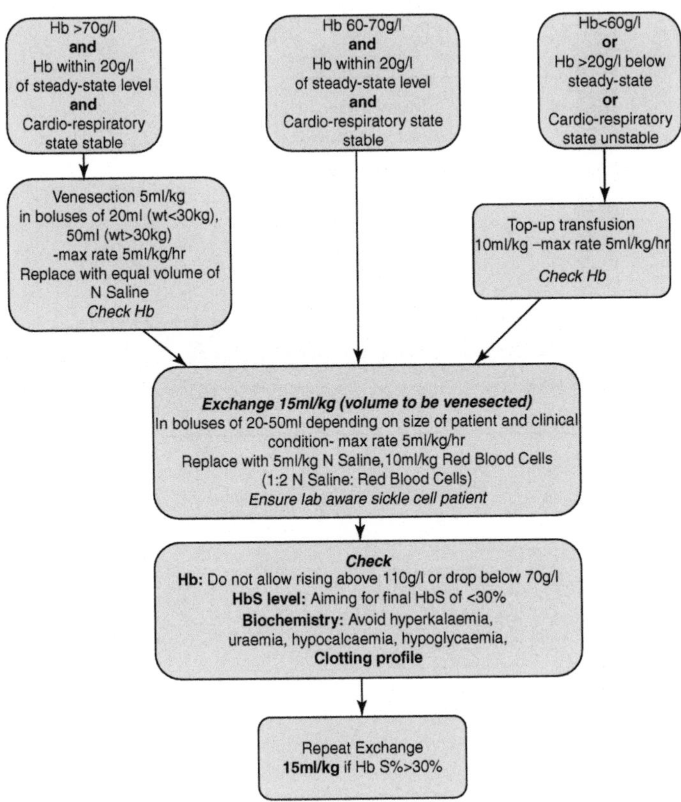

J. Howard, P. Telfer, *Sickle Cell Disease in Clinical Practice*, In Clinical Practice, DOI 10.1007/978-1-4471-2473-3,

Adult

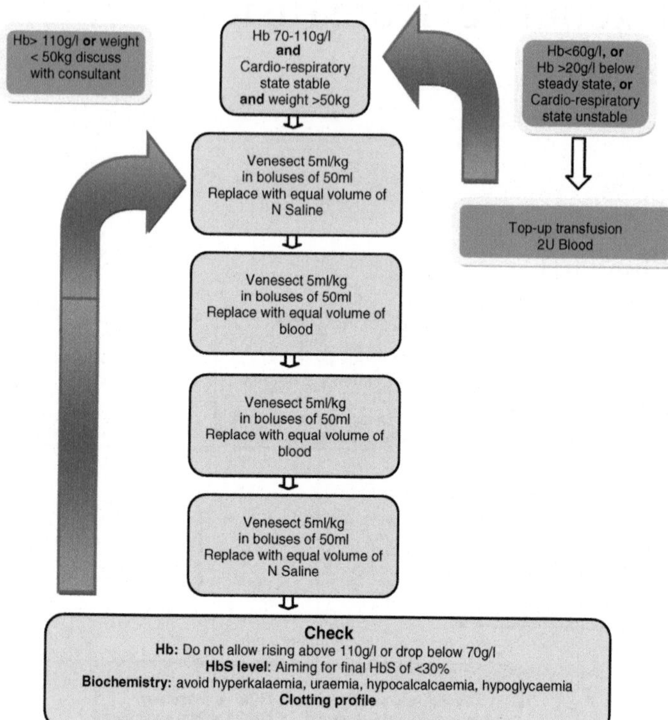
Hb> 110g/l **or** weight < 50kg discuss with consultant
Hb 70-110g/l **and** Cardio-respiratory state stable **and** weight >50kg
Hb<60g/l, **or** Hb >20g/l below steady state, **or** Cardio-respiratory state unstable
Top-up transfusion 2U Blood
Venesect 5ml/kg in boluses of 50ml Replace with equal volume of N Saline
Venesect 5ml/kg in boluses of 50ml Replace with equal volume of blood
Venesect 5ml/kg in boluses of 50ml Replace with equal volume of blood
Venesect 5ml/kg in boluses of 50ml Replace with equal volume of N Saline
Check
Hb: Do not allow rising above 110g/l or drop below 70g/l
HbS level: Aiming for final HbS of <30%
Biochemistry: avoid hyperkalaemia, uraemia, hypocalcalcaemia, hypoglycaemia
Clotting profile

Appendix 5: Annual Review Proforma

This proforma is based on the fields of the National Haemoglobinopathy Registry (NHR) and the data from here can be transferred into the NHR. Alternatively data can be entered directly on the internet forms of the NHR.

Name of reviewer: ____________________

Date of Annual Review:

About the patient:

Patient name: ________________
Hospital no: ________________

Date of birth:

Height: ---------------------cm

Weight: ---------------------kg

Spleen Size: ---------------------cm

Blood Pressure: ____________________mmHg

Oxygen Saturations: ____________________%

Centre Change in this Review Period: Yes ☐ No ☐

Number of Emergency (A&E or urgent day care) attendances (IN LAST 12 MONTHS): ☐
Number of Hospital Admissions (IN LAST 12 MONTHS)

Have they had a transfusion (IN LAST 12 MONTHS): Yes ☐ No ☐

Does the patient have an emergency care plan: Yes ☐ No ☐

Has the patient had any red cell antibodies: Yes ☐ No ☐

Have they fathered/mothered a child in this review period: Yes ☐ No ☐
If yes, outcome...
C section, Live birth, C section/live birth, ND, Preterm baby less than 36 weeks, Spontaneous miscarriage, Therapeutic abortion **(please circle)**

J. Howard, P. Telfer, *Sickle Cell Disease in Clinical Practice*, In Clinical Practice, DOI 10.1007/978-1-4471-2473-3,

Complications in this review period: (please circle)

Acute chest syndrome
Bone problems i.e. AVN, osteopenia, osteoporosis, other (**specify**)
Chronic Hepatitis C
Gallstones
HIV
Leg Ulcers
Multi organ failure
Osteomyelitis
Other (**please specify**)
Other bacteraemia
Parvovirus
Pneumococcal infection
Pulmonary hypertension
Renal failure
Severe septicaemia
Sickle retinopathy
Splenic sequestration
Stroke
TIA

Complication date(s): ____________________

Complication Continued: Yes ☐ No ☐

Comments:

Transfusion in this review period:

Transfusion Type	Start Date	End Date	Therapy continued	Total Estimated Transfusion Units in this Review Period	Comments
Long term transfusion Programme exchange					
Long term transfusion programme top up					
New alloantibody					
Transfusion exchange					
Transfusion top up					

Vaccinations in this Review Period:

Given in last 12 months or since last annual review whichever is longer.

Vaccination	Date Vaccine Given	Date Vaccine next due
Haemophilus		
Hepatitis B		
Influenza		
Meningitis + Hib (Menitorix)		
Meningitis group C conjugate		
Pneumovax		
Prevenar		
Other		

Investigations in this review period:

Investigation details	Date	Result
Audiometry		
Bone profile		
Brain MRI/MRA		
Creatinine		
Echocardiogram		
Ferritin		
FSH/LH		
Glucose Tolerance Test		
Liver function		
Mean Haemoglobin Untransfused		
Microalbuminuria		
Oestrogen (for females)		
Ophthalmology		
PTH		
Sleep study		
Steady state (untransfused)		
Testosterone (for males)		
Thyroid		
Virology serology – HepB, HepC, HIV		
Vitamin D		

Specialist Imaging:

Imaging	Date/result
Ferriscan Date:	
Cardiac T2' result (ms):	
Cardiac T2' date:	
Liver T2' Results (ms):	
Liver T2' date:	

Medications in this Review Period:

(I.e. over the last 12 months)
Give Date started/stopped if new med or discontinued. If long term med (patient was on it prior to last annual review) tick 'medication continued' box.

Medication	Date started	Date stopped	Medication continued	Comments
ACE Inhibitor				
Bisphosphonate				
Folic acid				
Hydroxycarbamide				
Other (**specify**)				
Penicillin V				
Vitamin D				

Iron Chelation in this review period:

Iron chelation type	Date started (if known)	Date stopped	Iron chelation continued	Comments
Combined Desferrioxamine + Deferiprone				
Deferasirox				
Deferiprone				
Desferrioxamine				
Other (**specify**)				

Operations in this Review Period

Operation	**Date of operation (if known)**	**Comments**
Adenotonsillectomy		
Hip replacement		
Laparoscopic Cholecystectomy		
Orthopaedic		
Other (**specify**)		
Retinal surgery		
Splenectomy		

Bone marrow transplant:

Transplant outcome	**Transplant start date (if known)**	**Transplant end date**	**Transplant continued**
Death			
Other (**specify**)			
Rejection			
Severe grade 3 or 4 GVH			
Successful Engraftment			

Any other comments:

Management plan:

Date set: Date completed:

To do Action: *Insert pain plan and action points from consultation.*

Index

J. Howard, P. Telfer, *Sickle Cell Disease in Clinical Practice*, In Clinical Practice, DOI 10.1007/978-1-4471-2473-3,